CHRIS COOPER

Breast Cancer:
The Shared Struggle

Table of contents

Dedication

To everyone who has played a significant role in my journey through breast cancer, this book is dedicated to you.

First and foremost, I express my deepest gratitude to the incredible women and men who shared their personal stories with me. Your strength and resilience have inspired me beyond words, and I hope this book honours your courage.

To my friends, though you were physically far, your messages and encouragement gave me the strength to face my diagnosis and the challenges that followed. Your love, even from afar, made an immeasurable difference in my darkest moments.

I extend my heartfelt appreciation to the dedicated medical professionals and staff who guided my treatment with expertise and compassion. From the doctors and nurses to the support staff who made every visit easier — your kindness had a profound impact on my journey. You are the unsung heroes who offer hope and strength when uncertainty looms.

To the community of cancer survivors, thank you for reminding me I am never alone. Together, we form a powerful network that transcends individual experiences, creating an unbreakable bond of support.

This book is also dedicated to all those fighting breast cancer and other forms of cancer. Your courage in the face of adversity inspires me every day. You are not just statistics or stories; you are warriors, each with a unique journey filled with moments of fear, strength, and resilience.

To the remarkable women I met along the way — those who shared their stories, offered words of encouragement, and showed me that vulnerability is not weakness but a reflection to our collective strength — your bravery taught me that in unity, there is power. In sharing our struggles, we uplift one another.

Lastly, to the medical professionals and support staff who devote their lives to caring for cancer patients, your compassion and expertise have touched the lives of many, including my own.

This book is my tribute to all of you. Your stories, unwavering support, and compassion have shaped my path, and I will forever be grateful.

Introduction

In life, we often believe we have a clear path ahead — setting goals, dreaming big, and making plans. But sometimes, life throws unexpected challenges that force us to reevaluate everything we thought we knew. For me, that moment came with a breast cancer diagnosis. It was an experience that not only changed my life but also reshaped my understanding of strength, vulnerability, and community.

Breast cancer is typically thought of as a women's disease, but as a male survivor, I learned firsthand how isolating it can be to navigate a diagnosis that isn't widely understood or discussed in men. My journey through surgeries and recovery has shown the power of resilience, but it also highlighted the importance of awareness, education, and support for all who are affected by this disease.

Why Did I Write This Book?

Now at 46 years old, seven years after my surgery, I still wake up in pain, reliving the events, the surgeries, and the long road to recovery. The memories resurface, each time delving deeper into the details that shaped my experience. Writing this book has been my way of making sense of that pain and reaching out to others who may feel isolated in their struggles.

I want readers to know they are not alone. By putting my story into words, I aim to heal—both myself and those who may find solace in these pages. This journey is not just about my past; it's about the resilience we all possess and the connections we can forge through shared experiences. As I reflect on my life and the challenges I have faced, I hope to inspire others to confront their own battles with courage and determination.

This book is in no way intended to bring fear. Its purpose is to educate, offer support, and foster hope for anyone affected by breast cancer. I want readers to know that healing is possible, even when the journey feels overwhelming. By sharing the raw reality of my experience, I hope to reach those who may feel isolated or misunderstood, and offer them a sense of solidarity.

As a male breast cancer survivor, I also want to challenge the misconceptions surrounding this disease. Breast cancer affects men too, and yet it remains a topic shrouded in stigma and silence. Through this book, I hope to raise awareness about male breast cancer, shed light on the unique challenges men face, and show that this is not just a women's issue — it is a human issue.

Purpose of the Book

The purpose of this book is multifaceted. First and foremost, it aims to educate and raise awareness about male breast cancer, a subject too often overlooked. By sharing my personal journey, I hope to shed light on the unique challenges men face and break down the stigma surrounding this diagnosis.

This book also serves as a source of support and solidarity for anyone touched by cancer, regardless of gender. I want readers to understand that they are not alone. Cancer's emotional and physical toll can feel isolating, but within these pages, I hope to offer stories that reflect the shared experiences of many. Together, we can create a dialogue that fosters understanding, compassion, and hope.

Additionally, this book is a tribute to the incredible women I met along my journey. Their resilience, courage, and strength inspired me every single day, reminding me that we are united in this battle, no matter our gender.

Through practical advice, emotional insights, and personal anecdotes, my hope is that this book empowers readers with knowledge and hope. I believe that by sharing our battles, we can strengthen the bonds between us and encourage meaningful conversations about health, awareness, and support. We are all in this together, and together, we are stronger.

Chapter 1

The Diagnosis That Changed Everything

My Initial Reaction

For ten long years, I chased answers. What began as a nagging pain grew into a persistent discomfort that felt impossible to ignore. No matter how much I tried to articulate my symptoms—how the pain intensified, how it began to resemble the size of a plum—my concerns seemed to fall on deaf ears. Doctors in both the UK and France brushed me off, attributing my discomfort to benign conditions. They suspected a cyst, yet they never pursued a deeper investigation. To them, I was merely a healthy-looking man with no apparent issues; my symptoms were dismissed as fabrications of an anxious mind.

This experience was profoundly frustrating. I felt trapped in a body that was speaking to me, yet the medical professionals I turned to for help failed to acknowledge its cries for attention. I began to doubt myself, questioning whether my pain was real or if I was indeed overreacting. I fought a silent battle, one that pitted my instincts against the scepticism of those sworn to protect my health. Each visit to the doctor chipped away at my confidence, leaving me feeling increasingly isolated and vulnerable.

Finally, after years of relentless pursuit, a breakthrough came. A doctor, after hearing my story and examining my condition, agreed to perform a biopsy. I remember the day vividly: the sterile smell of the hospital, sharp and clinical, mingling with the faint scent of antiseptic. Bright lights overhead felt almost blinding, casting harsh shadows that seemed to mirror my anxiety. As I lay on the examination table, a cold sweat broke out on my brow, my heart racing in anticipation. I was filled with a tumultuous mix of hope and fear—hope that this procedure would finally provide the answers I had long sought, but fear of what those answers might reveal.

The wait for the results felt agonizing. Each day stretched into an eternity as I replayed every moment in my mind, filled with questions that gnawed at me. Friends and family tried to reassure me, but their words felt distant, echoing in my mind as I focused on the unknown. I often found myself staring out the window, lost in thought, wondering how I could possibly prepare for whatever news awaited me. I imagined every scenario: what if it was benign? What if it wasn't?

Three weeks later, the day finally arrived. The sun shone brightly, almost tauntingly, as I made my way to the doctor's office. My hands trembled slightly as I sat in the waiting room, the silence punctuated only by the rustling of magazines and the ticking of the clock. I glanced at the faces around me, each person with their own battles, and felt an overwhelming sense of solidarity.

When my name was called, I took a deep breath and walked into the consultation room alone. There was no nurse to accompany me, and the emptiness of the space amplified my anxiety. The doctor entered shortly after, her expression serious, lacking any warmth or compassion. She sat down, and I could feel my heart pounding in my chest, each beat echoing in my ears.

"Your biopsy results are back," she said flatly. "I'm sorry to inform you that it shows a cancerous tumour."

The weight of those words crashed down on me, and for a moment, the room spun. It felt surreal, as if I were watching a scene unfold in a movie rather than living it. My mind raced: "Oh gosh," I thought, "it has been inside my body for so long. How long do I have to live?" The questions flooded in, each one heavier than the last.

The doctor continued with her explanation—details about the stage, treatment options, next steps—but her words felt clinical and distant. I struggled to absorb the information, feeling as though I was in a fog. All I could focus on was the gravity of the diagnosis, the stark reality that my life was about to change irrevocably.

I left the office that day with a mix of fear and determination. Though the path ahead was uncertain, I realized I had a choice: to fight back with everything I had.

In that instant, a torrent of emotions engulfed me—shock, disbelief, anger, and an overwhelming sense of urgency. How had it come to this? How could I have been left in the dark for so long? The frustration of those lost years surged through me, mingling with an anxiety that was both paralyzing and profound. I was overwhelmed by the realization that a part of my life had been consumed by a disease I had been fighting to understand for so long.

Time seemed to warp in that moment. Questions raced through my mind: Would I have to endure lengthy treatments? What would my future look like? Would I be able to continue my life as I knew it? I felt as if I were standing at the edge of a precipice, peering into an uncertain abyss. The fear of the unknown loomed large, and I struggled to find a foothold in this new reality.

Yet amid the chaos of emotions, a flicker of resolve began to ignite within me. This diagnosis, as devastating as it was, became a catalyst for change. I realized that I could no longer remain passive in my journey; I had to take control of my health and my narrative. I made a promise to myself that I would not let this disease define me, but rather let it fuel my fight for survival and understanding.

As I began to navigate this uncharted territory, I sought to learn everything I could about my condition. I reached out to support groups and connected with others who had faced similar battles. I immersed myself in the stories of survivors, drawing strength from their experiences.

This chapter of my life was not just about my diagnosis; it was about awakening a profound awareness of the shared struggles faced by all cancer patients, regardless of gender. My journey had begun, and while it was fraught with challenges, it was also filled with opportunities for connection, education, and advocacy.

The journey ahead would not be easy, but it was one I was now ready to embrace. I would advocate for myself, raise awareness, and honour the resilience of those I met along the way. I was determined to ensure that no one else would have to endure the years of silence I had faced, that no one else would be dismissed or doubted. This was just the beginning, and I was ready to face whatever lay ahead. As the reality of my diagnosis settled in, a whirlwind of emotions continued to swirl within me. I was inundated with thoughts about what this would mean for my friends and my life as a whole. Would I be able to fulfil my responsibilities? Would I be able to continue working, or would I have to lean on others for support? Questions raced through my mind like wildfire, each more daunting than the last.

What if I couldn't handle the treatment? Would I be a burden to my friends, the only support system I had? How would they cope with my illness? Would they still see me as the person I used to be, or would I become defined by my diagnosis? I couldn't help but wonder: without family to rely on, who would be there for me during the darkest moments?

The uncertainty loomed large. What if the treatment didn't work? What kind of future awaited me? I found myself grappling with fears not just about my health, but about my place in the world—my sense of belonging, my identity, and my ability to maintain the connections that meant so much to me.

In this sea of questions, I felt both lost and determined. I had to find a way to navigate this uncharted territory, not only for myself but for the friends who stood by me.

The gravity of cancer is not just in the physical toll it takes, but in the psychological burden it imposes. I found myself grappling with the notion of mortality. How long had this tumour been silently growing inside me? Had it already spread? The concept of time became increasingly elusive, and the urgency of my situation made every moment feel precious. I became acutely aware of the fragility of life, a feeling that lingered long after I left the doctor's office.

In the days that followed, I immersed myself in research about breast cancer. I discovered that, while it predominantly affects women, men are not immune. The statistics were startling, yet the stigma surrounding male breast cancer was even more shocking. Many people are unaware that men can develop this disease, leading to a profound sense of isolation for those diagnosed. It became clear to me that I had not only a personal battle to fight, but also a mission to advocate for awareness and understanding of male breast cancer.

I didn't reach out to others for support or seek solace; instead, I navigated this journey alone. The absence of guidance left me to my own devices, amplifying my feelings of solitude. I pored over countless articles, studies, and personal accounts, feeling both empowered and overwhelmed. While I longed for connection, I also recognized the importance of educating myself.

As I learned about the struggles and triumphs of those affected by this disease, I realized that even in my isolation, I could still find strength. Every day felt like a mix of hope and anxiety. I began to prepare for the appointments that lay ahead, mentally steeling myself for discussions about treatment options. Would I undergo surgery? Would I need chemotherapy or radiation? Each potential path felt daunting, yet I recognized that knowledge was power. I wanted to equip myself with as much information as possible to make informed decisions about my health.

My conversations with healthcare professionals became more pointed. I was no longer just a passive recipient of information; I became an active participant in my care. I asked questions that had once felt too daunting. I advocated for myself in a way I had never done before, pushing back against the dismissals of the past. This newfound determination to take charge of my health was both empowering and liberating.

In this period of my life, I began to understand the importance of vulnerability. While society often equates vulnerability with weakness, I discovered it to be a source of profound strength. Sharing my fears, my hopes, and my experiences became a form of catharsis. It allowed me to connect more deeply with others, fostering a sense of community and shared purpose.

As I prepared for the journey ahead, I made a commitment to embrace every moment. I decided that I would not allow fear to dictate my choices. Instead, I would focus on living fully, cherishing the moments I had, and using my voice to advocate for those who felt unheard. This period, while marked by uncertainty and fear, was also an opportunity for growth, connection, and empowerment.

I understood now that my diagnosis was not just a personal battle; it was a call to action. It was a chance to shed light on the realities of breast cancer, to create awareness, and to contribute to a dialogue that included everyone affected by this disease. In that spirit, I felt a sense of purpose igniting within me—a determination to transform my experience into something meaningful.

As I moved forward, I carried with me the knowledge of those who had faced similar challenges, knowing that even in my solitude, I could create a ripple effect of change. This was only the beginning, but I was ready to face whatever lay ahead with courage and conviction. The journey would be challenging, but I was committed to fighting not just for myself, but for all who shared in this struggle. As the days turned into weeks, the weight of my diagnosis continued to shape my daily life. I found myself oscillating between moments of determination and waves of despair.

Each new appointment felt like a step into the unknown, a path laden with uncertainties. I would sit in waiting rooms, surrounded by other patients, each grappling with their own battles, and I realized how the shared experience of cancer created an unspoken bond. Despite our differences, we were all seeking understanding, hope, and healing.

During those waiting periods, I often reflected on how long I had lived with my symptoms. I thought about the years of pain I had dismissed, the countless times I had been told I was fine, and the frustration of not being taken seriously. It became evident that my journey was not just about facing cancer; it was about confronting a system that had failed to listen. My experience was a stark reminder of the importance of advocacy—not only for myself but for others who might find their voices silenced by scepticism.

Each consultation brought new information that felt both empowering and overwhelming. I learned about stages, treatment options, and the importance of a multidisciplinary approach to care. I was fortunate to connect with an oncologist who not only understood the complexities of male breast cancer but also took the time to listen to my concerns. Their approach helped me feel more secure, providing clarity in a landscape that had once felt chaotic and frightening. I came to realize that finding the right healthcare team was crucial; they were not just treating a disease but a person with hopes, fears, and dreams.

As I learned to navigate the complexities of my diagnosis, I found myself reevaluating my priorities. Without friends around to share the journey, the realization that life is fleeting urged me to appreciate simple moments—savouring a meal, listening to the quiet sounds of nature, or taking time for reflection. I started to see beauty in the everyday, understanding that these moments were gifts, heightened by my experience with cancer. Living became an act of defiance against the disease that sought to take so much from me.

Moving through the early stages of my diagnosis, I began to recognize the power of storytelling. I understood that sharing my journey could not only provide me with catharsis but also offer hope to others. With no one close to confide in, I felt an urgency to document my experiences, creating a narrative that encompassed both the struggles and the triumphs. Writing became my way of connecting with others who might feel as isolated as I did, reminding them that they are not alone and that their stories matter.

Every night, I would sit down with my journal, pouring my thoughts and emotions onto the pages. It became a therapeutic practice, allowing me to process the rollercoaster of feelings that came with my diagnosis. I wrote about my fears, my hopes, and the lessons I was learning along the way. In doing so, I found clarity, purpose, and a newfound strength that surprised me. I was no longer just a patient; I was an advocate, a storyteller, and a survivor in the making.

Ultimately, my diagnosis marked the beginning of a profound journey—not just through illness but toward self-discovery and advocacy. As I moved forward, I realized that my experience with breast cancer was not merely about fighting a disease; it was about embracing life in all its complexity.

In the face of uncertainty, I found empowerment. I was ready to fight, ready to connect, and ready to embrace this new chapter of my life with open arms. This was just the beginning, and while the road ahead might be fraught with challenges, I knew I wouldn't be walking it alone.

Understanding Male Breast Cancer

As I began my journey through treatment, one of the most crucial steps was to understand the condition that had dramatically altered my life: male breast cancer. This disease is often overshadowed by its more common female counterpart, leading to a lack of awareness and understanding among both the public and medical professionals. My quest for knowledge not only helped me make informed decisions about my health but also ignited a passion to raise awareness about this often-misunderstood condition.

The Basics of Male Breast Cancer

Breast cancer occurs when cells in the breast tissue begin to grow uncontrollably, forming a tumour. While it is widely considered a women's disease—affecting approximately one in eight women—men can also develop breast cancer, though at a much lower rate. In fact, about 1 in 833 men will be diagnosed with breast cancer in their lifetime. This rarity often leads to misconceptions, causing many to overlook the possibility that men can be affected, which can delay diagnosis and treatment. Although men have less breast tissue than women, they still possess a small amount of glandular tissue, making breast cancer possible. Most male breast cancers originate in the ductal tissue, where abnormal cells can form. In women, these ducts would normally transport milk, but in men, the tissue has no such function. However, cancer can still develop here, and like in women, tumours can become invasive, spreading to nearby tissues or even metastasizing to distant parts of the body. Male breast cancer often goes unnoticed or is diagnosed late due to a lack of awareness. By understanding that breast cancer doesn't discriminate by gender, we can encourage earlier detection and ensure that men receive the same life-saving treatments as women.

Risk Factors and Early Detection

Understanding the risk factors associated with male breast cancer was vital for me. Several factors can increase a man's likelihood of developing this disease, including age, family history, genetic mutations (such as BRCA2), and conditions that affect hormone levels, such as Klinefelter syndrome.

Klinefelter syndrome is a genetic condition in which a male is born with an extra X chromosome, resulting in a XXY chromosome pattern rather than the typical XY. This condition can lead to hormonal imbalances, specifically lower levels of testosterone, which may increase the risk of developing breast cancer. Men with Klinefelter syndrome often experience other symptoms, such as reduced fertility, breast tissue enlargement (gynecomastia), and learning difficulties. Men with a family history of breast cancer—either maternal or paternal—should be particularly vigilant, as hereditary factors can play a significant role in their risk. By recognizing these risk factors, I understood the importance of early detection and proactive health measures.

Unfortunately, the lack of awareness surrounding male breast cancer often leads to late diagnoses. Many men do not recognize the symptoms or feel comfortable discussing them, resulting in delays in seeking help. Common signs to watch for include lumps or masses in the breast tissue, changes in the shape or contour of the breast, discharge from the nipple, or skin changes like redness or dimpling. Understanding these symptoms is crucial for early detection and improving outcomes.

The Stigma and Silence

One of the most significant barriers to awareness is the stigma associated with men having breast cancer. Many men may feel embarrassed or ashamed to discuss their symptoms, fearing ridicule or disbelief. This stigma can lead to silence, compounding the challenges of an already difficult diagnosis. I realized that breaking this silence was essential not only for my own healing but for raising awareness among others.

In conversations with fellow patients and survivors, I learned that many had experienced similar feelings of isolation. They often described the bewilderment of being diagnosed with a disease that was widely considered to be exclusive to women. It became clear that fostering open dialogue about male breast cancer was critical to dispelling myths and encouraging more men to seek help.

Transforming Fear into Action

Understanding male breast cancer became more than just a personal endeavour; it transformed into a collective mission. By educating myself and others, I could help change perceptions and empower men to be proactive about their health. I hoped to inspire other men to recognize symptoms, seek medical attention, and not shy away from discussing their experiences.

As I continued to navigate my treatment journey, I became increasingly passionate about transforming my fear and uncertainty into action. I wanted to ensure that no one else would have to endure years of being unheard or dismissed as I had. I understood that awareness could save lives, and I felt a deep responsibility to be a part of that change.

Chapter 2

Alone in the Waiting Room

Experiences in a Predominantly Female Environment

Navigating a predominantly female environment during my cancer journey was both enlightening and challenging. The waiting room for my first oncology appointment felt like entering a world that was simultaneously familiar and foreign. It was filled with women, each grappling with their own stories of strength and struggle, and the air was thick with unspoken emotions. While I encountered compassion and solidarity, I also experienced moments of disconnect. Conversations often revolved around shared experiences of femininity and motherhood, leaving me feeling somewhat out of place. Nevertheless, I learned the value of empathy and discovered common ground in vulnerability. The strength and resilience of the women around me inspired me, reminding me that, although our battles differed, the emotional landscapes we navigated shared profound similarities. In that waiting room, I felt a mix of fear, anxiety, and isolation, and I realized that my struggle was intertwined with theirs, highlighting the power of connection even in such a daunting space. As I took a seat among the rows of chairs, I noticed the palpable tension in the air. The room was a tapestry of emotions, where laughter and tears intertwined, creating an atmosphere thick with unspoken understanding. I observed the women around me: some were accompanied by supportive friends or family members, while others sat alone, their expressions reflecting a complex blend of hope and despair. Yet, I felt like an intruder in this sacred space. Despite the shared experience of cancer, my discomfort as the only man in the room amplified my feelings of loneliness. I was there to confront a life-altering diagnosis, yet my struggle seemed to take on a different dimension through the lens of a female-centric experience.

The anxiety in that waiting room was palpable. Conversations were hushed, and a collective tension loomed over everyone. I could hear snippets of discussions—treatment plans, side effects, and upcoming surgeries. Each word carried a weight of uncertainty. It struck me that these women were confronting their mortality in raw and immediate ways. I, too, was in a battle for my life, yet the camaraderie typically found in shared struggles felt elusive.

As I sat there, my mind raced with questions. Would I be subjected to the same painful treatments they faced? Would my journey mirror theirs, or would I find a different path? The anxiety bubbled up within me, leading to a series of "what ifs" that spiralled out of control. I thought about the potential for surgery, chemotherapy, and the fear of the unknown. I yearned for a connection, for someone who could understand the unique challenges I faced as a male breast cancer patient.

In that waiting room, I also noticed the unspoken resilience of the women around me. Despite their fear, there was an underlying strength that radiated from them—a collective determination to fight against a disease that sought to take so much from them. I admired their bravery, yet it made my own fear feel more pronounced. How could I, a man in this predominantly female space, connect with their experiences while still feeling my own struggle?

As my name was called, I felt a mix of relief and dread. I was grateful to be moving forward, yet I couldn't shake the feeling of isolation that had clung to me. The nurse led me through a door that separated the waiting room from the clinical world, and I turned back for a moment to take in the scene. I realized that while I might be alone in this particular fight, I was not truly alone. Each woman there was navigating her own journey, and in that shared struggle, there was a sense of unity that transcended gender.

In the examination room, the atmosphere shifted once again. I faced my oncologist, who was knowledgeable and compassionate. I began to articulate my fears and concerns, feeling a little more at ease in this clinical environment. Yet, the waiting room lingered in my mind. I reflected on how that space had encapsulated the complexity of cancer— fear intertwined with hope, isolation blended with community.

Moving forward, I knew I would carry the weight of those experiences with me. I was determined to break the silence surrounding male breast cancer, to reach out and connect with others who might feel similarly alone. My time in that waiting room, though difficult, would serve as a catalyst for change. I would not allow my experiences to go unheard; instead, I would seek to foster a sense of solidarity that included everyone affected by breast cancer, regardless of gender.

In sharing my journey, I hoped to bridge the divide that I had felt so acutely. I wanted to remind others—men and women alike—that vulnerability does not diminish strength. We all face battles that may feel isolating, but by coming together, we can create a community of support, understanding, and hope. My experience in the waiting room had opened my eyes to the complexities of this shared struggle, and I was determined to ensure that no one else would have to navigate it alone. As I settled into the sterile environment of the examination room, the memories of the waiting room lingered. I could still hear the soft murmurs of conversation and the occasional bursts of laughter that tried to pierce through the heaviness of fear. The juxtaposition of life and illness seemed almost surreal. How could laughter coexist with the gravity of cancer?

Sitting there, I reflected on the stories I had overheard—tales of resilience, of women who had faced unimaginable challenges and emerged stronger. I felt a twinge of envy for the connections they seemed to share, a bond forged in the fires of adversity. Their experiences were different from mine, but I began to realize that the essence of their journeys—grappling with fear, navigating treatment, and holding onto hope—was universal.

Yet, my reality as a man with breast cancer often felt distinct. I pondered how society has constructed narratives around gender and illness, often portraying women as the primary victims of breast cancer while rendering men invisible. This invisibility deepened my sense of isolation. It was crucial to me that my voice was heard—not just for my own sake but for the countless men who may suffer in silence, feeling their struggles overlooked or minimized.

As the doctor entered the room, I steeled myself for the conversation ahead. Their demeanour was warm, but the clinical nature of the environment reinforced my anxiety. I felt as if I were stepping into a script where I was the only male character, surrounded by an audience of women. The doctor began discussing my diagnosis, the treatment options available, and the next steps. I listened intently, but my mind drifted back to the waiting room, where a different kind of dialogue unfolded—one filled with shared fears, unguarded emotions, and heartfelt encouragement.

The disparity between the room I was now in and the waiting room filled with women made me acutely aware of my unique position. I longed for a space where I could openly express my fears, share my story, and feel the solidarity of others who understood what it meant to navigate this uncharted territory. I needed to find my voice among the noise, to contribute to a conversation that included men without overshadowing the experiences of women.

After my appointment, I made a conscious decision to reach out to those women I had encountered in the waiting room. I wanted to connect, to share not just my story but also the common threads that united us. In doing so, I hoped to create a dialogue that transcended gender—a narrative that embraced all individuals affected by breast cancer, highlighting the strength and resilience inherent in our shared struggles.

With newfound determination, I began to explore online support groups and forums where I could engage with others facing similar challenges. I sought out organizations that focused on male breast cancer awareness, eager to contribute my voice to the collective effort. I learned that many men were hesitant to share their experiences, often feeling isolated and unsure of where to turn. By connecting with these individuals, I hoped to foster an environment where vulnerability was celebrated, and silence was broken.

In the weeks that followed, I attended a support group specifically tailored for cancer patients. Walking into the room, I felt a mix of apprehension and hope. I was again entering a predominantly female space, but this time, I was armed with the knowledge that our struggles were interwoven. As I sat down, I introduced myself and shared my diagnosis. To my surprise, I was met with warmth and understanding. Women in the group responded with encouragement, and I felt the walls of isolation begin to crumble.

One woman, in particular, spoke about her journey with breast cancer, emphasizing how important it was to share experiences across genders. She expressed gratitude for my presence, stating that every voice mattered, and together, we could amplify the message that breast cancer knows no gender. This recognition validated my feelings and underscored the importance of fostering connections within our community.

I started to understand that while my experiences as a man might differ in some ways, the emotional landscape we navigated was remarkably similar. Fear, hope, loss, and resilience wove through all our stories, creating a tapestry of shared humanity. I began to embrace the idea that our individual battles could unite us in ways I had never anticipated.

The more I participated in these discussions, the more I realized the power of storytelling. It was a way to bridge the gaps, to create understanding where there had been misunderstanding. By sharing my story, I could help dismantle the stigma that often-surrounded male breast cancer and encourage other men to find their voices. I envisioned a future where no one would have to endure their journey in silence, where all experiences—male or female—would be acknowledged and honoured.

My time in that waiting room, while filled with fear and anxiety, had ultimately catalysed a transformation. It sparked a desire to advocate for awareness and understanding, to ensure that every individual affected by breast cancer could find community, support, and solidarity. As I stepped out of that examination room, I was no longer just a patient navigating the complexities of cancer. I was part of a movement—a chorus of voices determined to break the silence and foster a shared understanding of the human experience in the face of adversity.

Moving forward, I was committed to embracing my journey, to sharing my story, and to standing alongside the women I had encountered in that waiting room. Together, we could create a dialogue that honoured all experiences, weaving our stories into a powerful narrative of hope, resilience, and collective strength. No one should have to face their battle alone; it was time to bridge the divide and lift each other up, united in our shared struggle against breast cancer. As I continued to attend appointments, the waiting room became a familiar backdrop to my evolving understanding of breast cancer. Each visit felt like a continuation of a journey that was unfolding not just within me but within the lives of those around me. I began to observe the little rituals that unfolded in that space: women exchanging comforting smiles, sharing tissues, or engaging in hushed conversations about the treatments they were undergoing. Each interaction carried a weight, as if they were all part of a shared pact to navigate this labyrinth together.

Yet, despite the camaraderie among the women, I couldn't shake the feeling of being an outsider. I would often hear discussions about hair loss, the emotional toll of mastectomy, or the complexities of family dynamics when a loved one is diagnosed. I listened intently, often finding myself wishing I could contribute to these conversations. But how could I express my fears and experiences without seeming out of place? It was a delicate dance—wanting to connect while grappling with the fear of intruding.

In those moments of quiet observation, I also recognized the profound loneliness that cancer can impose. The waiting room, despite being filled with people, often felt isolating. I saw women lost in thought, staring blankly at the walls, their minds racing with worries about the future. Their faces were a canvas of hope tinged with anxiety, revealing the duality of their existence: fighting against a formidable foe while yearning for normalcy.

I couldn't help but reflect on my own internal struggles. The fear of the unknown loomed large. What if the treatment didn't work? What if the cancer returned? These questions echoed in my mind, exacerbating the sense of isolation. It was a surreal experience to be surrounded by people who understood the gravity of illness, yet feel disconnected from their shared narratives. I longed for a space where I could voice my fears, yet the waiting room remained a realm of silent battles.

One day, as I sat waiting for my name to be called, I overheard a group of women discussing their upcoming chemotherapy sessions. The laughter that accompanied their conversation struck me as both genuine and heartbreaking. They were creating bonds in the face of adversity, turning a daunting experience into moments of shared laughter. I admired their strength, but I also felt a pang of sadness. Why was I, a man facing a similar fate, not able to engage in that same light-heartedness?

In a moment of courage, I decided to introduce myself. I stood and approached a small group of women who seemed open to conversation. "Hi, I'm a male breast cancer patient," I said, my voice steady despite the apprehension swirling inside me. "I just wanted to say that I admire how you all support each other. It's really inspiring."

To my surprise, they welcomed me warmly. They shared their own stories and expressed gratitude for my presence, reinforcing that my experiences were just as valid. One woman, in particular, spoke about her brother, who had faced breast cancer years ago. She shared how the family had struggled to understand his experience and how much she wished there had been more visibility for male patients.

This moment felt transformative. For the first time, I realized that by sharing my story, I could help foster connections. It was a reminder that we are all navigating our own paths, and there is power in vulnerability. The walls I had built around myself began to crumble, allowing for authentic conversations that bridged the gender divide.

As I continued to visit the clinic, I made it a point to engage with others in the waiting room. I learned about their journeys and shared mine in return. Each interaction deepened my understanding of the collective struggle we all faced, regardless of gender. I began to see the similarities in our fears, hopes, and desires for healing.

I also started to notice a shift in how I perceived my own experience. Instead of viewing my diagnosis as a solitary journey, I began to see it as part of a larger narrative—a tapestry woven from the stories of everyone in that room. It dawned on me that by engaging with these women, I was not only helping myself but also contributing to a broader dialogue about breast cancer.

One afternoon, as I sat quietly in the clinic, I reflected on my journey. I hadn't shared my story with anyone, but I found myself observing the people around me—women talking softly about their experiences, exchanging supportive smiles. Though I remained silent, I realized how important it was for male voices to be part of these conversations. Breast cancer wasn't just their battle; it was mine too. The isolation I felt in that moment deepened my resolve to bring awareness to male breast cancer, even if I chose to walk this path alone. That day, as I left the clinic, a new sense of purpose emerged. The waiting room, once a place filled with anxiety and a sense of otherness, had become a quiet reminder of the shared struggles we all face, regardless of gender. My journey wasn't just about fighting cancer—it was about challenging the silence, even if I didn't speak up directly. I understood that my role could be just as powerful in solitude, breaking barriers through quiet resilience.

As I walked out of the clinic, I felt a weight lift from my shoulders. The waiting room had taught me lessons about resilience and the unseen strength in facing something without sharing it. I was no longer just a patient; I was becoming an advocate in my own way—determined to raise awareness for men like me, bridging the gap between genders in the shared struggle against breast cancer.

Building Connections

As time passed, I began to realize that carrying the weight of my experience alone was more difficult than I had anticipated. The silence, once a protective shield, started to feel heavy and isolating. I thought I could navigate this journey by relying solely on research and inner strength, but the emotional toll of facing cancer without sharing my burden became undeniable. Every appointment and each new piece of information felt like another layer of isolation. I understood that while solitude had its strength, it could also be suffocating. The mental and emotional weight of remaining silent was just as exhausting as the physical toll of the disease itself. It wasn't until I tentatively began to open up, first to my healthcare team and later to a few trusted individuals, that I experienced a significant shift. Speaking about my diagnosis and my feelings of isolation felt like releasing a long-held breath. I no longer needed to carry this alone. Slowly, I realized that connection—sharing my story, no matter how uncomfortable or vulnerable it made me feel—had a power all its own. It was magical in a way I hadn't expected. By giving voice to my struggle, I not only lightened my own burden, but I also found strength in the shared humanity of those around me. They, too, had their fears and battles, and though our journeys were different, the act of speaking up bridged the gap between us.

Building connections transformed my perspective. I saw that cancer wasn't just a solitary fight; it was a collective experience. Sharing the weight of the journey didn't make me weaker; it made me stronger.

The more I opened up, the more I understood the value of community and advocacy. The magic lay not only in the act of speaking up but in the empathy and understanding others extended toward me. It reminded me that my voice mattered, and that in breaking the silence, I was no longer alone.

I found that sharing my experience didn't need to be limited to others with cancer. When I allowed myself to speak to friend and acquaintances—people who didn't necessarily understand the medical specifics of my journey—I discovered a surprising and profound sense of connection. They understood pain, fear, and the universal need for support. By opening up, I realized that everyone, in their own way, has faced battles that shaped their lives. It wasn't about having the exact same experience; it was about sharing the human condition of facing hardship and uncertainty. Talking to those who didn't have cancer but had their own struggles reminded me that vulnerability is universal. Whether someone had faced illness, loss, or personal challenges, there was always common ground in the emotional landscape of navigating life's difficulties. In sharing my journey, I let others in on what I had been carrying alone for so long. The responses were different than I expected—not clinical or rooted in shared illness, but deeply empathetic and genuine. These conversations revealed that my fears, frustrations, and hopes resonated beyond the confines of a diagnosis. It became less about cancer specifically, and more about learning how to live with uncertainty, face fear head-on, and find strength in unexpected places.

What truly surprised me was how much lighter I felt with each conversation. I didn't need to detail every aspect of my medical battle; it was enough to simply express what I had held inside for so long. Opening up gave me the courage to be vulnerable and honest, and in return, I found support in places I hadn't anticipated. Speaking to people who didn't share my exact experience was still magical, allowing me to connect on a deeper level of human resilience. It reminded me that strength isn't just in facing the storm alone; it's in the courage to let others in, no matter where they're coming from.

Chapter 3

The Emotional Toll

Navigating Fear and Vulnerability

The diagnosis of breast cancer marked the beginning of a profound emotional journey—one that would lead me through a labyrinth of fear, vulnerability, and unexpected resilience. The initial shock of my diagnosis was a heavy weight that settled in my chest, making it difficult to breathe. It was as if I had been plunged into an unfamiliar world where uncertainty reigned, and every day brought new challenges.

The Weight of Fear

Fear, in its many forms, became an ever-present companion. The fear of the unknown loomed large, casting a shadow over my thoughts. Questions swirled endlessly in my mind: How advanced is the cancer? What treatments will I need? How will this affect my life as a whole? These questions often felt overwhelming, creating a mental fog that made it difficult to focus on anything other than the looming spectre of my diagnosis.

At first, my fear was mainly focused on the immediate—worries about treatment options and my physical health. But as the reality of my situation began to sink in, I found myself grappling with deeper, more existential fears. These thoughts created a cycle of anxiety that felt impossible to escape.

In the waiting rooms of hospitals and clinics, I would often catch glimpses of other patients' faces— some etched with worry, others marked by resignation. We shared an unspoken understanding; we were all navigating this tumultuous sea of fear. It became clear that fear was a universal experience, one that transcended gender, age, and background.

Vulnerability: A Double-Edged Sword

In the midst of my emotional turmoil, I discovered something unexpected: vulnerability is a double-edged sword. While it is often seen as a weakness, it can also be a source of profound connection and healing. My first instinct was to shield myself from it, to lock away my fears and present a brave face to the world. I told myself it was better this way—better to pretend I was fine, better not to worry my friends. Deep down, though, I feared that if I let my true emotions surface, I would be nothing but a burden.

It started the day I received the news from my doctor. The word "cancer" lingered in the air long after I hung up, and suddenly, the future seemed like a vast, dark void. That night, I sat on my bed staring at the ceiling, my thoughts racing. What if the treatment didn't work? What if I lost my hair, my strength— myself? The fear spiralled into anxiety about everything, even mundane things like my career and finances. I wanted to talk to someone, but the thought of unloading my anxiety felt selfish.

Still, there came a moment when I couldn't keep it all inside anymore. I called a close friend, my voice shaky. I remember saying, "I don't want to scare you, but I'm terrified." Expecting hesitation, I was instead met with a long, soft silence. Then, in a quiet voice, she said, "Me too." She wasn't scared of cancer, but she spoke of her own fears—how uncertain life had become, how fragile her plans for the future now felt. She admitted she had been lying awake at night, anxious about her job, her relationships, and whether she was making the right choices. In that moment, I realized we were both carrying heavy burdens, ones we had kept hidden for too long.

The more I shared, the less isolated I felt. Anxiety still creeps in—I won't pretend it doesn't—but it no longer holds the same power over me. In speaking my fears out loud, they became less like shadows looming over me and more like companions, shared and understood. In that sharing, I began to feel a small, but real, sense of peace. And in the midst of my storm, that peace felt like a gift.

Embracing Emotional Waves

As I navigated my journey, I came to understand that emotions are not linear; they ebb and flow like the tides. One moment, I would feel hopeful, envisioning a future beyond cancer, and the next, I would be overwhelmed by despair, haunted by the thought of potential loss. This emotional rollercoaster was exhausting, yet I learned to embrace it as part of my experience.

I found solace in writing. Journaling became a therapeutic outlet where I could express my thoughts and feelings without judgment. Through the written word, I could explore the depths of my fear and vulnerability, transforming them into something tangible. This process of externalizing my emotions allowed me to confront them rather than suppress them.

In those moments of despair, I often turned to the stories of the women who inspired me. Their journeys reminded me that while fear is a natural response to uncertainty, it does not have to dictate my path. Each woman had faced her own emotional battles, and their resilience became a guiding light during my darkest moments.

The Role of Support Networks

Throughout my journey, I learned the vital importance of support networks. The friends who rallied around me became my pillars of strength. Their unwavering presence offered a sense of security amidst the chaos. When my fears felt insurmountable, they provided reassurance, helping me navigate the emotional toll of my diagnosis. Though I didn't actively seek support at first, I now understand how essential it is, especially for those without close family or friends. Facing a diagnosis like cancer can leave you feeling emotionally unstable and overwhelmed. In such moments, reaching out for support—whether through counselling, support groups, or community resources—is crucial. No one should go through this alone, and having people to lean on can make all the difference in finding stability and hope during such a challenging time.

Finding Empowerment in Vulnerability

As I continued to navigate the emotional landscape of my diagnosis, I began to reframe my understanding of vulnerability. Instead of viewing it as a weakness, I recognized it as an opportunity for growth and empowerment. By acknowledging my fears, I was able to confront them head-on, transforming them into sources of motivation.

I started to set small goals for myself, whether it was participating in a community event or engaging in self-care practices. Each achievement, no matter how small, served as a reminder of my strength. I learned that vulnerability could be a powerful catalyst for change, pushing me to step outside my comfort zone and embrace life more fully.

The Healing Journey

Ultimately, navigating fear and vulnerability became integral to my healing journey. I discovered that it is possible to coexist with fear while still finding joy and meaning in life. By embracing my emotions and allowing myself to be vulnerable, I found a sense of authenticity that deepened my relationships and enriched my experience.

The emotional toll of breast cancer is undeniable, but within that toll lies the potential for growth. I learned that it is okay to feel fear, to acknowledge vulnerability, and to seek support. These experiences are part of the human condition, and by embracing them, I could foster a deeper connection to myself and those around me.

Embracing the Full Spectrum of Emotions

As I reflect on my journey through fear and vulnerability, I realize that this emotional landscape is not a place to fear but a realm to explore. It is a space where we can discover our inner strength, connect with others, and ultimately, find healing. The emotional toll of cancer may be heavy, but it is also a teacher, guiding us toward a deeper understanding of ourselves and our capacity for resilience.

In sharing my story, I hope to encourage others to navigate their own emotional landscapes with courage and authenticity. By embracing vulnerability and seeking connection, we can transform our fears into a source of strength, fostering a sense of community that uplifts us all. Together, we can face the emotional toll of cancer, supporting one another as we journey toward healing and hope.

The Complexity of Grief

As I found out that surgery would be the first step to remove the tumour, I began to grasp the depth of grief that would accompany my diagnosis. It wasn't just the fear of what I might lose, but also the mourning of the life I once knew. The grief was complex, manifesting in unexpected ways—it wasn't just about my health, but about losing my sense of normalcy, my independence, and the carefree days that suddenly felt out of reach.

Each phase of treatment brought its own form of loss. After the surgery, I grieved the loss of my physical strength, and the emotional toll drained my energy. Simple tasks became monumental challenges, and I found myself longing for the vitality I had always taken for granted. This physical weakness was more than frustrating—it compounded my feelings of fear and vulnerability, creating a whirlwind of emotions that often felt impossible to untangle. Grief, in all its complexity, became a constant companion, making the emotional journey of healing as difficult as the physical one.

Emotions can be unpredictable, often shifting from one moment to the next. Some days, I would feel hopeful, buoyed by the support of friends. Other days, a wave of despair would crash over me, leaving me feeling adrift and lost. I learned to accept that this emotional rollercoaster was part of the journey.

During these low moments, I found solace in mindfulness practices. Meditation and deep-breathing exercises helped ground me in the present, allowing me to observe my feelings without judgment. Instead of trying to suppress or fight against my emotions, I learned to sit with them, acknowledging their existence and allowing them to flow through me.

Mindfulness taught me the importance of self-compassion. I began to recognize that it was okay to have bad days, to feel overwhelmed, or to cry. Each emotional ebb and flow was a natural part of my healing journey, a reminder that I was human and experiencing something profoundly challenging.

Chapter 4

Chapters of Courage: My Surgical Experience

Receiving a cancer diagnosis is often just the beginning of a journey filled with physical and emotional hurdles. When I first learned that surgery would be my primary treatment, I didn't fully grasp how much it would challenge me, not just physically but mentally as well. The fear of the unknown lingered, but the determination to fight back was strong. Still, once the initial shock wore off, I realized that the road ahead would be long, and it wasn't just about removing the tumour—it was about navigating a new way of living. The day of the surgery arrived, and while I'll delve into the specifics of the procedure later, what struck me most in those early days was the sheer weight of recovery. The physical toll was immediate. Tasks I had once taken for granted, like lifting my arms or even sitting up in bed, suddenly felt monumental. I remember lying there, staring at the ceiling, overwhelmed by the loss of independence. The pain was sharp and unrelenting at first, a constant reminder of how drastically things had changed. But more than the pain, it was the feeling of vulnerability that truly tested me.

At first, I felt frustrated by my body's limitations. I had always been strong, self-sufficient, and now even simple movements seemed impossible. But slowly, I learned to adjust. The key, I found, was setting small, achievable goals. One day, I would aim to walk a few steps around my room. The next, I would challenge myself to stretch a bit farther or lift my arms just a little higher. These small victories, though they seemed insignificant in the grand scheme of things, became the building blocks of my recovery. Each success—no matter how small—lifted my spirits and restored a sense of control in an otherwise uncontrollable situation.

In those early weeks, I also realized the importance of patience. I had always been someone who pushed through challenges, expecting my body to bounce back quickly. But surgery taught me a different kind of strength—the strength to be kind to myself, to recognize that healing isn't a race. It's a process that requires grace. I learned to listen to my body, resting when I needed to, and not feeling guilty for the days when progress seemed slow. There were emotional challenges too. The grief of losing a part of myself and adjusting to a new physical reality weighed heavily on me. It wasn't just about the surgery or the physical pain—it was the realization that my body would never be the same again. That sense of loss was difficult to process. But as I continued to heal, I found strength in resilience. Slowly but surely, I learned that recovery wasn't about returning to who I had been before—it was about embracing who I was becoming. This journey, though difficult, taught me to find balance.

Some days were filled with frustration, while others brought hope. And through it all, I discovered that healing, much like life, is rarely linear. It comes with its share of setbacks, but also moments of triumph. Those moments—however fleeting—were enough to carry me through.

As I reflect on my journey through cancer, there's one night that stands out vividly—a night that felt like the precipice of my new reality. It was a time filled with uncertainty and anxiety, a true nightmare in the making. In the hours leading up to my surgery, I was consumed by a whirlwind of emotions—fear, loneliness, and the weight of what lay ahead. This was no ordinary night; it was the night before everything changed. I will now share the details of that fateful evening, a night spent grappling with the unknown as I prepared to embark on a journey that would test my strength in ways I had never imagined. The hospital in Lyon had a reputation for specializing in cancer treatment, and my oncologist insisted it was the best place for my procedures. Because I had two procedures to undergo, I knew I needed the best care possible, but traveling there alone filled me with a quiet sense of dread. My journey began in Orléans, where I lived, and would take me nearly five hours away to Lyon, where I would face the first step in my fight against cancer.

I left Orléans in the late afternoon, dragging a small suitcase behind me as I navigated the city's tram system, my mind already a thousand miles away. From the tram, I transferred onto the first train to Paris, then from Paris to Lyon. As I sat by the window, watching the familiar scenery of Orléans fade away, I couldn't help but feel a pang of loneliness. The train's rhythmic clatter only amplified the thoughts swirling in my head. What would happen tomorrow? Was I really ready for this? I hadn't let myself fully absorb the reality of the surgery—of what it meant to have a tumour removed from my body. That night, though, as the train sped toward Lyon, there was no avoiding it.

By the time I boarded the second train, the sun had already dipped below the horizon. The once crowded train station had grown quiet, and I felt the weight of the evening pressing down on me. My second train ride was quieter and darker as I tried to lose myself in a book but couldn't manage to focus on the words. All I could think about was the procedure waiting for me on the other side. I remember looking at the other passengers and wondering what their lives were like, whether they, too, were heading toward some life-altering event. But their faces gave nothing away. I felt invisible in my own dread.

After two tube rides through the maze of Lyon's metro, I finally arrived at my hotel. It was a modest place—nothing fancy, just a bed and a bathroom. But that night, it felt like the loneliest room in the world. I checked in, dragging my suitcase behind me, and sank into the bed, staring up at the ceiling. Soon after, a migraine hit me—sharp and relentless, the kind that made it hard to think, let alone relax. I had no appetite for dinner, no desire to explore the city I had once loved to visit. I was here for one reason, and that reason filled every corner of my mind, leaving no room for anything else. That night, I hardly slept. Between the anxiety and the pounding migraine, I tossed and turned until the early hours of the morning. When the first hints of daylight filtered through the curtains, I reluctantly got up, knowing what the day ahead held. I had been instructed to scrub myself thoroughly with Betadine before leaving for the clinic. The smell filled the small hotel bathroom—sharp and medicinal—as I methodically washed, making sure every inch of my body was clean. The scrubbing felt like a ritual, a final preparation before the unknown. Afterward, I had to travel five kilometres to reach the private clinic, and though it wasn't far, the trip felt like an eternity. The taxi ride through Lyon's bustling streets was a surreal contrast to my inner turmoil. Life outside seemed to carry on as usual—people were going to work, walking their dogs, and laughing on sidewalks. But inside, I was a knot of tension, unable to shake the feeling that everything was about to change.

At the clinic, they administered a chemical injection designed to trace the lymph nodes that might be affected by the cancer. The nurse warned me to stay away from infants and pregnant women due to the radiation in the chemicals. That warning stuck with me, making me feel like a walking hazard, further isolating me from the world around me. As I sat in the sterile waiting room, I couldn't help but feel an overwhelming sense of vulnerability.

Finally, it was time. I was led into a stark white room, where I was handed a hospital gown and told to lie down on the bed. My head throbbed with the relentless migraine, and as I lay there, staring at the ceiling, the reality of the situation began to sink in. I was alone, far from home, about to undergo surgery that would alter my body and, possibly, my life. The loneliness was palpable. There were no friendly faces, no familiar voices. Just me, the sterile smell of the clinic, and the fear gnawing at the pit of my stomach. As I tried to steady my breathing, the anaesthesiologist came into the room, his face serious. He held a folder in his hands, flipping through my medical results. When he spoke, his tone was calm, but his words hit me like a punch to the gut. **"We can't proceed with the surgery,"** he said, his expression serious as he

held my gaze. "Your blood tests show an issue with clotting. It's too risky—you could bleed uncontrollably, leading to possible death on the table."

The words hung in the air, heavy and chilling. My heart raced as the stark reality of the situation sank in. **Bleed to death?** I had mentally prepared for countless possibilities that day—pain, anxiety, the arduous journey to recovery—but the notion of death had never crossed my mind. It felt like a scene ripped from a horror film, where the stakes had suddenly escalated beyond anything I could grasp. The weight of those words pressed down on me, amplifying my fear and vulnerability as I struggled to process what this meant for my future. I could barely process what he was saying when the door swung open again, and in walked my oncologist. Unlike the anaesthesiologist, he seemed eager to move forward. He sat at the edge of my bed and urged me to reconsider. "We've come this far," he said, his voice a mixture of persuasion and impatience. "The surgery needs to happen. We can monitor the bleeding."

But the thought of dying on the operating table terrified me more than the idea of postponing the surgery. My mind was spinning, caught between the oncologist's insistence and the anaesthesiologist's caution. Could I really go through with it, knowing the risk? In that moment, I felt utterly alone, forced to make a decision that could determine my fate. I refused. I wasn't willing to gamble with my life, not like this. They would need to run further tests, check my blood clotting issues, and I would have to wait. My oncologist sighed, clearly frustrated, but there was no convincing me. The idea of undergoing surgery with a potentially life-threatening complication was too much. They arranged for me to have more blood tests back in Orléans, and just like that, the surgery I had been dreading was put on hold.

As I left the clinic, the streets of Lyon seemed colder, the journey back to Orléans longer. The exhaustion, both physical and emotional, weighed heavily on me as I boarded the train. I wasn't sure what the future held, but one thing was clear: my journey with cancer had only just begun, and it would be filled with more uncertainty and difficult decisions than I could have ever imagined.

Five days after returning to Orléans, I got the call. My blood tests were clear—my blood clotting issues had been resolved, and the surgery was back on. The oncologist's voice was steady, almost routine, as if we hadn't already been through this. But for me, it was a gut punch. Here we go again. I packed my small suitcase once more, bracing myself for the journey I thought I'd already completed. The familiar exhaustion settled in as I caught the tram, then the train, heading back to Lyon. The same route, the same anxious anticipation, but this time the dread was quieter, dulled by repetition. I couldn't help but think about the injection waiting for me, the radioactive chemicals they'd put in my body again to trace the lymph nodes. The thought lingered—this time, more eerie than before—as I mentally prepared myself to feel like a walking hazard once more. The warning to avoid pregnant women and infants still echoed in my mind as I arrived at the hotel. The same hotel, the same modest room. It felt even smaller this time, the walls closing in on me as if they knew what was coming. I wasn't there to explore the city or find some comfort in the familiar streets. I was there to confront my fear again, head-on.

That night, I was given a tube of cream with clear instructions: apply it to your chest to remove any hair before surgery. The surgeons had made a point of it, but I wasn't focused. I was too tired, too anxious to think beyond the next few hours. So, I smeared the cream haphazardly, not really paying attention to where I was applying it. I just wanted to get it done and try to rest before the long day ahead. But as the night wore on, a sharp burning sensation began to spread across my chest. At first, it was a dull discomfort, but then it escalated into a searing pain. That's when I realized my mistake. I had gotten the cream too close to my nipples, and they were now burning, on fire with the same intensity as my growing anxiety. My chest throbbed, my nipples raw and stinging with every slight movement. The pain kept me awake all night, adding to the migraine of emotions I was already wrestling with. I tossed and turned, desperate for relief, but nothing helped. The throbbing was relentless, and it felt almost absurd— of all the things I was supposed to be preparing for, here I was suffering from careless use of hair removal cream.

By the time the first light of morning streamed through the curtains, I hadn't slept. The exhaustion was bone-deep, not just from lack of sleep but from the weight of everything looming ahead. My chest still burned, my nipples aching with every breath, but there was no time to dwell on it. The surgery was waiting, and I had no choice but to face it head-on. I made my way back to the clinic, my chest still tender and sore under my shirt. The same injection awaited me—the radiation chemicals coursing through my body, marking me once again as a walking hazard. I tried to shake the feeling, to focus on the surgery itself, but it lingered, an invisible burden I couldn't quite shrug off. As I walked through the clinic doors, that same sterile smell hit me, a reminder that this place would soon be the scene of one of the most important moments in my life. This time, though, there was no rush of panic, no overwhelming sense of doom. Instead, there was a strange calm, almost like acceptance. My chest burned, my mind was clouded with a thousand thoughts, but I had finally come to terms with one thing: this surgery needed to happen. There was no more delaying, no more running from it. The uncertainty was still there, gnawing at me, but I knew I had to go through with it. As they handed me the hospital gown once again, I slipped into it without complaint, the fabric resting uncomfortably on my still-burning chest. I lay down on the bed, closed my eyes, and took a deep breath. I didn't know what would happen next, but for the first time in days, I wasn't trying to fight the unknown.

The morning moved forward like clockwork, each moment pulling me closer to the operating table. After the usual pre-op formalities—signing consent forms, confirming my identity and the procedure—the door opened, and in walked the surgeons. I wasn't surprised; they had explained earlier that their involvement would be necessary due to the location of my tumour. It wasn't just any surgery to remove cancer—I would also need plastic surgery to reconstruct my chest.

The tumour's proximity to my right nipple made it impossible for the oncology team to remove it without affecting the surrounding tissue. To complicate matters, I also had gynecomastia—excess tissue in my chest—which added another layer of complexity to the surgery. The plastic surgeon would need to collaborate closely with the oncology surgeon to ensure my chest looked as normal as possible after the tumour was excised. This wasn't just about survival; it was also about preserving a sense of wholeness, making sure I didn't wake up looking like a stranger to myself.

The oncologist, a tall, soft-spoken man, explained the procedure again, though this time the details felt sharper, more direct. He and the plastic surgeon had made a decision: saving my right nipple was no longer an option. The tumour's location made it too risky. Both nipples would have to be removed. They would then use tissue from my left nipple to reshape and reconstruct both through a process called a nipple graft. "We'll remove the right nipple entirely," he said, his tone steady but firm. "Then, we'll reshape your left nipple and use it to recreate the appearance of both. The plastic surgery team will handle the grafting. While there's no guarantee of full sensation afterward, the goal is to restore as much of the natural look as possible."

His words, calm and measured, hit me like a punch. The reality of losing both nipples—regardless of the reconstruction—felt unsettling. This wasn't just about removing a tumour anymore; it was about living with a body permanently altered, bearing the visible scars of a fight for survival. As the plastic surgeon began marking my chest, he carefully traced where the incisions would be made, explaining how they would reattach the grafted tissue. Each stroke of the pen seemed to map out the parts of me I was about to lose. The lines felt more significant than just surgical markers—they outlined the changes my body would soon undergo. When the markings were complete, the plastic surgeon stepped back, his part in the process done for now. "After the tumour is removed, we'll come in for the reconstruction," he reassured me. "You're in good hands."

Moments later, the oncologist returned with a new sense of urgency, his eyes focused and determined. Unlike the plastic surgeon, his concern wasn't about aesthetics or reconstruction—it was about the tumour and removing it before it caused more harm. To him, this was a battle, and he was leading the charge. I nodded, the weight of his words pressing down on me. The tumour, which had seemed like a distant threat, now felt very real, like a foreign object sitting just beneath my skin, close to the nipple. I hadn't fully registered its presence until that moment, but now, with two surgical teams preparing to operate, the gravity of the situation was undeniable.

By the time the surgeons were done explaining everything, my chest was a canvas of black markings and planned incisions, each line representing a different phase of the operation. I felt like an anatomical diagram—every part of me mapped out for removal, reconstruction, and healing. The lines on my skin told a story of both destruction and renewal, of what cancer had already taken and what the surgeons would try to salvage. It was overwhelming, seeing my body reduced to lines and shapes, reduced to something that needed fixing. But I didn't have time to spiral into anxiety. The machine of surgery was already in motion, and I was simply being carried along by it. Before I could dwell on what the next hours might bring, they wheeled me out of the room and down the long hallway toward the operating theatre. The ceiling lights flashed overhead, one after another, as the gurney rolled beneath them, each light pulling me closer to the unknown.

As they wheeled me toward the operating room, the weight of it all began to settle in. This wasn't just a single surgery, not just the removal of a tumour—it was two surgeries. Two surgeons. One to save my life by cutting out the cancer, and the other to rebuild what the disease had tried to take from me. In the haze of my thoughts, I realized this wasn't a battle I was fighting alone. These surgeons, with their scalpels and sutures, were my allies in a war against my own body. And yet, I couldn't shake the loneliness that settled over me like a heavy blanket.

As the double doors of the operating room swung open, I was met with the sharp, sterile brightness of the lights. The room hummed with quiet efficiency—nurses moving with practiced precision, instruments gleaming under the intense light, machines blinking and beeping in readiness. It was an orchestrated chaos, controlled and purposeful, and yet, to me, it felt surreal. This was the place where my life, my body, would be irrevocably altered. They transferred me onto the operating table, the cold surface pressing against my back, a jarring contrast to the warmth of the gurney. My chest, still marked with the surgeon's ink, lay exposed under the bright lights, and for the first time, I felt the vulnerability of it all. The nurses moved around me, checking tubes and preparing the IV. Their faces were calm, unhurried, as if this were just another day for them, but for me, it was anything but routine.

The anaesthesiologist entered, the same man who had warned me about the blood clotting risks just days ago. His face was serious, but now there was a hint of reassurance in his eyes as he approached. He spoke softly, explaining that he would be putting me under, that soon I wouldn't feel anything at all. His words were meant to comfort me, but they only heightened my awareness of how close I was to the point of no return. As he prepared the anaesthesia, I stared up at the bright surgical lights, trying to steady my breathing. It was a losing battle. My mind was racing, replaying the morning's events over and over. The plastic surgeon's precise markings, the oncologist's stern words, the reminder that both my nipples would be removed and reconstructed, the thought of waking up with a body I no longer recognized. The stakes felt enormous. This was about more than just survival—this was about identity, about how I would piece myself back together both physically and mentally. The mask was placed over my face, and I inhaled deeply, the sterile scent of the operating room mingling with the cool rush of gas. I could hear the faint beeping of machines in the background, the sound growing distant as the anaesthesia started to take hold. The room seemed to blur around the edges, the lights above me becoming softer, less glaring. My thoughts, once spinning out of control, began to slow, as though someone had turned the volume down on my anxiety. "Just breathe," the anaesthesiologist said, his voice calm and steady, guiding me through the process. "In and out. You'll drift off soon."

I focused on my breathing, feeling the cool air fill my lungs, then release in a slow, deliberate exhale. The fear, the uncertainty, and the weight of everything faded into the background, as if a curtain was slowly being drawn over my consciousness. My last conscious thought before I slipped under was simple, but profound: **I hoped I would wake up whole.** Then, as the anaesthesia fully kicked in, the world around me dissolved into darkness, and I closed my eyes.

When I began to wake, it was as though I were floating up from the depths of a dark, endless ocean. The world felt distant, muffled, and for a moment, I wasn't sure if I was awake or still caught in some foggy dream. My body felt heavy, unresponsive, as if it belonged to someone else. Everything was soft, blurry, like I was swimming through thick fog. Slowly, sensations started creeping back—first, a dull ache in my chest, then the dryness in my throat. I tried to swallow but felt a strange resistance. It took me a second to realize what it was: a tube. There was a tube in my throat, stiff and uncomfortable, pushing against the back of my mouth. Panic flickered in the corner of my mind, but my body was too sluggish to react.

A soft voice broke through the haze. I couldn't quite make out the words, but the tone was gentle, reassuring. My eyes fluttered open, the harsh fluorescent lights of the recovery room stabbing at my vision. The world was still hazy, the outlines of people and objects fuzzy, but I could see a nurse standing beside me, her face half-covered by a surgical mask. She was speaking again, her voice low and calm, telling me it was time to remove the tube. The nurse's hands moved with practiced precision as she gently gripped the tube. A wave of discomfort rolled through me as she began to pull. The sensation was strange, invasive—like something foreign was being dragged out from the depths of my throat. I gagged, my body's natural reflex kicking in, but I was too weak to do much more than squirm slightly. The tube slid out slowly, scraping against the rawness of my throat, and with one final pull, it was gone. I gasped for air, my first instinct to breathe deeply now that the obstruction was gone. My throat burned, dry and raw, as though I had been breathing in sand. Every breath felt rough and laboured, but at least I could breathe on my own again. The nurse was still there, her voice a quiet hum, telling me to take it slow. "Breathe, nice and easy," she said, and I tried to follow her instructions, focusing on the steady rhythm of my own breath. As the fog in my head began to lift, the room around me came into sharper focus. The white walls of the recovery room, the sterile smell of antiseptics, the quiet beep of monitors surrounding me—it was all real. I was awake, I was alive. The surgery was over. But then, the ache in my chest began to grow. It wasn't just the soreness of a normal surgery—it felt deeper, like something had been taken from me. I shifted slightly, my movements sluggish, and a fresh wave of discomfort rolled over me. I remembered everything now. The tumour. The double surgery. My nipples. I tried to move my arm to reach for my chest, to feel what was left, but the nurse gently stopped me. "Don't move too much just yet," she said softly. "Everything went fine. You're in recovery now." Her words were meant to soothe, but I couldn't help the swirl of emotions rising in me. My mind was racing, my body still too numb to fully register what had just happened. I couldn't feel my chest—not really. It was just a dull, throbbing ache under the layers of bandages. I wanted to touch it, to know what was left, to know how much of me was still there, but I was too weak, too groggy to do anything but lie there. I tried to speak, to ask questions, but my throat was too dry, my voice a raspy whisper. The nurse understood without me saying a word.

As the minutes ticked by, I could feel the anaesthesia wearing off, leaving me more and more aware of my body. The soreness in my chest became more prominent, a dull reminder of what I had just gone through. My mind kept going back to the surgery, to the tumour they had removed, and to my chest—the part of me that had been altered in ways I couldn't yet see or fully understand. I was alive. That was the most important thing. But the reality of what came next— the healing, the scars, the new version of myself I would have to face—was just beginning to sink in.

The first time I tried getting out of bed, it was like my body no longer belonged to me. I had been lying still for hours, the post-surgery haze slowly wearing off, when I felt the need to go to the toilet. With great effort, I swung my legs over the edge of the bed. My head swam immediately, a heavy, dizzying fog clouding my thoughts. Every inch of my body protested, especially my chest, a dull, persistent throb radiating from the freshly stitched wounds. I gripped the bed rails for support, breathing through the wave of nausea that suddenly hit me. My legs felt weak, almost rubbery, but I had convinced myself that I could manage. I took a shaky step forward, reaching for the IV stand beside me. But as I moved, my vision started to blur, a tunnel of darkness closing in from the edges. Panic surged in my chest—I wasn't going to make it. I barely had time to call for a nurse before everything went black. I came to on the cold, hard floor, confused and disoriented. A sharp sting radiated from my chest as I realized what had happened—I'd collapsed. The room around me was a whirl of activity as nurses rushed in. One of them, her face full of concern, knelt beside me, speaking in calming tones I could barely hear over the pounding in my head. I could feel them lifting me gently, carefully manoeuvring me back onto the bed. "Don't try to stand up so soon," one of the nurses said as they propped me back against the pillows. "Your body's been through a lot. Take it easy." I nodded weakly, too exhausted to respond. Every movement felt laboured, as if I were swimming through molasses. My chest throbbed with every breath, a constant reminder of what I had just endured. The nurses fussed over me, adjusting the IV, checking my vitals. The exhaustion was so intense that I felt myself drifting in and out of consciousness, the edges of the world blurring into a soft haze once again.

Later that day, the nurses came in to check on my wounds. I knew this moment was coming, but the anticipation of it filled me with dread. I lay still, my body tense, as they slowly peeled back the bandages. The smell of antiseptic filled the air, sharp and medicinal, mingling with the sterile atmosphere of the hospital room. I couldn't bring myself to look. The idea of seeing my chest—of seeing the damage, the scars, the parts of me that had been cut away—was too much. I kept my eyes firmly closed, focusing on the steady sound of my breathing as the nurses worked in silence. Their hands were gentle but firm as they cleaned the incisions, their touch clinical but careful. I felt the cool sting of disinfectant on my skin, but I forced myself not to flinch. I could feel the tension in the room, a kind of quiet, focused concentration as they assessed the wounds, their murmurs of approval or concern barely audible over the blood rushing in my ears. Still, I didn't dare open my eyes. I wasn't ready to face what lay beneath those bandages. Not yet. It wasn't long before I noticed one of the nurses growing quiet, her movements slowing as she examined the right side of my chest. Her brow furrowed as she leaned in closer, her fingers gently probing the skin. I could hear her call for another nurse, and the subtle shift in her voice told me something was wrong. My heart began to race, a sinking feeling settling deep in my gut. "There's some necrosis here," she said softly, but the words struck me like a hammer. Necrosis. My skin was dying. The next moments passed in a blur of quiet conversation between the nurses, their voices tense and serious. I lay there, eyes still shut, my mind racing with possibilities. What did this mean? How bad was it? What would they need to do?

Less than 24 hours after the surgery, the plastic surgeon came in, his face serious but calm as he explained what had happened. "We were as cautious as we could be," he said, his voice steady but with an undercurrent of tension. "But a small artery was cut during the procedure, and it's causing issues with the blood flow to that part of your chest. If we don't flush out the blood and improve circulation, the skin will continue to necrose." The words hit me like a punch to the gut. The careful balance they had tried to maintain during the surgery had failed. I would need to go back into the operating room, and soon. Otherwise, the skin on my chest—already fragile, already fighting to heal—would die completely. I felt gutted, like the ground had been ripped out from under me. I had known this surgery would be difficult, that complications were always a risk, but hearing it now, so soon after everything I'd already been through, was devastating. My chest, which had already been marked, cut, and reconstructed, was now in danger of losing more. As the surgeon explained the procedure, I felt the fear creep up my spine. I wasn't even a day into my recovery, and I was already facing another trip back under the knife. "You'll need to go back in," the surgeon said gently, as though he could sense the fear rising in me. "We need to make sure the blood flow is restored, or the damage will spread." I nodded, but inside I was terrified. The thought of another surgery, of being cut open again, of the very real possibility that my body might not heal the way it should, filled me with dread. How much more could my chest take? How much more could I take?

As they prepared to schedule the second operation, I felt a deep sense of helplessness wash over me. No matter how cautious the surgeons had been, no matter how careful their planning, things had still gone wrong. Now, the only thing standing between me and the loss of my skin was another surgery, another set of incisions, and more uncertainty. I lay back in bed, the words of the surgeon still echoing in my mind, feeling the weight of it all settle heavily in my chest. I had thought the worst was behind me, but now, I wasn't so sure. As they prepped me for the second surgery, I found myself back in the cold, sterile environment of the operating room, staring up at the bright overhead lights. The familiar antiseptic smell filled my nostrils, and the sounds of surgical instruments clinking together echoed faintly in the background. It was happening again. My chest, barely healed, was about to be cut open for a second time. My mind was racing, a swirling storm of fear and uncertainty. I couldn't shake the thought—what if this time, it didn't go as planned? What if they couldn't stop the necrosis? What if I woke up and there was more damage? My chest felt fragile, like a delicate piece of fabric on the verge of tearing, and now I was being sent back under the knife with no guarantee of success.

As they prepared to administer the anaesthesia, the same anaesthesiologist from the first surgery approached me, his face partially obscured by the surgical mask. Despite his calm, professional demeanour, I could sense that he remembered me. He must have seen countless patients come and go, but something in his eyes told me that he hadn't forgotten the anxiety I carried with me the first time I lay on that operating table. And now, here I was again. He paused for a moment, looking down at me with a mixture of concern and understanding. His eyes met mine, and in that brief second, it was as if he could see straight through me, straight into the fear that I was desperately trying to hide. I didn't need to say anything—my heart was pounding, and my chest felt tight as I tried to keep my breathing steady. But I knew he could tell. He placed a gentle hand on my arm, leaning in slightly. His voice was low, calm, and reassuring, but not in a way that felt rehearsed. He wasn't just going through the motions; he was trying to reach me, to ease the fear he saw so clearly in my eyes. "I know this is difficult," he said softly, his words cutting through the haze of my panic. "But you're in good hands. We'll take care of you, just like we did before." I tried to nod, but my throat felt tight. The weight of what was about to happen pressed down on me, heavy and suffocating. He could sense it, too. "You're strong. You've already come this far," he added, his hand still resting gently on my arm. "We'll get you through this."

There was something about the way he said it, the quiet conviction in his voice, that made me believe him—if only for a moment. I took a shaky breath, trying to push the fear aside as the anaesthesiologist prepared the IV. His hand was steady as he adjusted the needle, and I watched, almost in slow motion, as he began to push the anaesthetic into the tube. The last thing I remember was his voice, calm and steady, as he spoke to me again. "Close your eyes," he said softly. "We'll see you on the other side." I did as he said, letting the heaviness of the anaesthetic take over, my body slowly surrendering to the numbing darkness. My eyelids fluttered, and then everything faded to black.

The surgery, thankfully, went well. When I woke up, the nurses' voices were softer, their movements more relaxed, and the plastic surgeon came by with a nod of reassurance. "We managed to flush out the blood," he said, offering a small, tired smile. "The skin should heal properly now." Then the oncologist came in with the results of my lymph nodes, explaining that three had been removed during the surgery. He reassured me that my life expectancy had just gone up, as the cancer hadn't spread anywhere else. "The right nipple we removed wasn't contaminated with cancer, but we couldn't take the risk of keeping it." He also informed me that I would not need radiotherapy or chemotherapy. Relief flooded through me, but it was quickly overshadowed by the pain and exhaustion that had settled deep into my bones. My chest, though no longer under immediate threat, felt like it had been torn apart and pieced back together. The recovery would be long.

I had expected to be out of the hospital within a couple of days, but complications stretched my stay longer than planned. I was weak, my body sluggish from the two surgeries in quick succession, and the nurses kept a close watch on the incisions. Every dressing change was an ordeal, and I still couldn't bring myself to fully look at my chest. The scars were too fresh, the trauma too recent. Eventually, though, the hospital decided I was stable enough to go home. But with my extended stay, plans for my friend to pick me up had fallen apart. She had commitments she couldn't delay any longer, and by the time I was finally discharged, she was no longer able to drive to Lyon to take me back to Orléans. I was left on my own. I had never felt so vulnerable. The idea of navigating two trains and the journey home—like this—was daunting, to say the least. My body, battered and bandaged, felt fragile, and every movement was a painful reminder of what I had just endured. The medical team tried to reassure me, offering advice on how to travel safely, but I knew it was going to be an uphill battle.

The taxi picked me up from the hospital and dropped me off at the train station. I had packed light when I first arrived in Lyon, but even dragging that small suitcase behind me now felt like climbing a mountain. My arms trembled from the effort, and the strain on my chest was immediate, sharp, and unforgiving. I gritted my teeth and pushed through the station, willing myself to keep going. But halfway across the platform, I couldn't do it anymore. My chest felt like it was splitting open, and my legs were shaking uncontrollably. I stopped in my tracks, the suitcase handle slipping from my fingers. The weight of it was too much. I couldn't carry it any longer. I stood there, looking down at my suitcase, helplessness and frustration washing over me. I had come so far, endured so much, and yet here I was, defeated by something as simple as luggage. I boarded the train, my chest still throbbing, the weight of exhaustion pressing down on me. Every bump and jolt of the train felt like a shockwave through my body, and all I could do was sit there, staring blankly out the window as the countryside blurred past. My only focus was getting home. The second train felt even longer than the first. By then, I was on autopilot, barely aware of my surroundings, just one step away from collapsing into the seat entirely. The journey that had seemed difficult before surgery now felt like an impossible task, but somehow, I made it. When I finally arrived back in Orléans, I was numb—physically and emotionally. I had made it through the surgeries, survived the journey home, but the reality of what I had endured and the long road ahead of me was just beginning to settle in.

The recovery was far harder than I had anticipated. Once I was back home in Orléans, the full weight of what I'd been through hit me. The relief of surviving two surgeries quickly gave way to the harsh reality of healing on my own. My chest was a mess of stitched-together skin, painful and fragile. Every breath, every slight movement, reminded me of how broken my body had become. The simplest tasks—getting out of bed, standing up, reaching for a glass of water—felt monumental. And then, of course, there was the loneliness. I had no one close by to help with the basics: no one to cook for me, go grocery shopping, or help me clean up and handle the chores. My friends, the few who had stayed in my life throughout this ordeal, were scattered—some abroad, others in distant cities. The one friend I had lived about 50 kilometres away, I couldn't bring myself to ask for help. Something in me hesitated. Was it pride? Shame? Or just the fear of being a burden?

It was hard to pinpoint what exactly held me back. A part of me didn't want to appear weak or needy. I had fought through so much, endured the surgeries, faced death twice, and now, asking for something as simple as a home-cooked meal felt like admitting defeat. But another part of me wondered if I was just ashamed. Ashamed that, despite everything I had been through, I couldn't manage alone. I should have been stronger. I should have been able to take care of myself—or at least, that's what I told myself. The days were long. Some mornings, I'd wake up with a deep, aching pain that spread through my chest, and I couldn't bring myself to get out of bed. I would just lie there, staring at the ceiling, listening to the quiet hum of the outside world. Life was happening out there—people were going about their days, going to work, living—but inside, I felt trapped in my own isolation.

I had enough pre-packaged meals to last me the first few days, but once they ran out, I was faced with the grim task of figuring out how to feed myself. I'd stare at the empty fridge, wondering where the energy would come from. Eventually, I'd drag myself to the nearest supermarket, but the walk there and back felt like a marathon. My chest throbbed with every step, and the weight of the bags pulled on my healing scars, making me wince in pain. I'd return home, exhausted, collapsing into a chair before I even had the energy to cook. I thought about calling my friend, the one who lived just 50 kilometres away. It wasn't far, but it felt like an insurmountable distance. I kept telling myself, *Don't bother them. They have their own lives to deal with. Why would they come all this way just to help me?* But deep down, I knew it wasn't about them; it was about me. I didn't want to admit that I needed someone. I didn't want to say out loud that I couldn't handle it all by myself. Maybe it was shame. Or maybe it was fear—the fear of what needing help really meant. That I wasn't invincible. That after everything I had survived, I was still vulnerable. I still don't know if it would've been shameful to ask for help. Maybe it was pride. Or maybe it was just me, still struggling to accept that, even after the battle with cancer, I didn't have to do everything on my own.

The recovery wasn't just lonely; it was brutal. Every day, I had to face the mirror and try not to wince at what I saw—bruises, scars, and the painful reminder of everything my body had been through. The nurses who came to treat my wounds didn't sugarcoat it either. One of them, a kind woman who tried to offer comfort but couldn't quite hide her reaction, looked me over one day and said, "You look like you've been hit by a truck." Not exactly what you want to hear. But she wasn't wrong. My chest, bruised and swollen, looked like a battlefield. The hematoma had spread from my chest all the way down to the bottom of my back, a deep purple-black mass of bruised tissue. The discoloration was so intense that at times, I could barely tell where the surgery scars ended, and the bruising began. Every move I made felt like my body was tearing apart from the inside. The nurse's words stuck with me long after she'd left. I didn't need anyone to tell me how bad I looked—I could feel it with every breath. But hearing it out loud was different. It was a brutal confirmation of just how far my body had fallen. I wasn't just healing; I was recovering from a trauma that had spread deeper than I could've ever imagined. Each day, the nurses came by, gently cleaning the wounds and reapplying fresh bandages. Despite their care, I couldn't bring myself to look directly at the incisions. My chest—once mine—now felt like something else entirely. I could feel the stitches tugging at my skin, the constant soreness, but I avoided actually seeing it. I wasn't ready. The sight of my body so broken, so altered, was too much to bear. I felt disconnected, like the person lying there wasn't fully me anymore. One of the nurses noticed how I avoided looking, and she told me it was normal—everyone reacts differently to seeing their post-surgery body. But her words, meant to comfort, didn't reach me. I couldn't shake the image of my body bruised and torn.

As you can imagine, or perhaps grasp from the details of the surgeries I went through, I had to relive each instant while writing this—and it wasn't the first time. I am scarred for life, both in body and mind, but I feel at peace because I survived. These scars, though painful, are symbols of my endurance, reminding me that I've faced what seemed impossible and emerged on the other side. While the memories and the pain remain, I now understand the importance of reaching out. I use that strength to help others going through cancer because I understand the pain and loneliness they face—even if I didn't fully recognize it at the time. I no longer need to prove my strength—to myself or anyone else—but I can share my journey to offer hope and support to those who need it most.

Chapter 5

Strength Beyond Gender

Redefining Masculinity and Vulnerability

In a society where masculinity is frequently associated with stoicism, strength, and emotional restraint, my journey through breast cancer forced me to confront and challenge these deeply ingrained beliefs. As I navigated the physical and emotional toll of the illness, I realized that the traditional ideals of masculinity—rigid self-reliance and an aversion to vulnerability—no longer served me. Instead, I discovered that true strength lies not in suppressing emotions or facing struggles in isolation, but in embracing vulnerability, seeking support, and allowing myself to be open in the face of adversity. This experience reshaped my understanding of what it truly means to be strong, revealing a profound connection between vulnerability and authentic strength, where courage is found in honesty and resilience comes from acceptance.

The Initial Conflict

When I received my diagnosis, I found myself grappling with conflicting emotions. On one hand, I was a man facing a disease that many associate predominantly with women; on the other, I was acutely aware of societal expectations surrounding male strength. Initially, I felt pressure to maintain a facade of bravery and resilience. I worried about how my diagnosis would be perceived—not just by others, but by myself. Was I still "manly" if I openly expressed fear or sought support?

In the early stages of my treatment, I noticed how societal norms influenced my behaviour. I often minimized my emotions, hesitating to voice my fears or concerns. I worried that acknowledging my vulnerability would somehow undermine my identity as a man. This internal conflict created a tension that was hard to reconcile, leaving me feeling isolated in my experience.

Challenging Societal Norms

The journey through breast cancer served as a powerful catalyst for challenging societal norms surrounding masculinity. Traditionally, men are taught to be stoic, to "man up" in the face of adversity, and to avoid expressing emotions. However, cancer has a way of dismantling these rigid expectations, forcing us to confront the reality that vulnerability is a part of life—regardless of gender.

Lessons from Female Patients

The women I met throughout my journey were particularly instrumental in reshaping my views on strength and vulnerability. They openly discussed their battles, fears, and triumphs, offering insights that challenged my preconceived notions about gender roles. Their stories often emphasized the importance of community, emotional expression, and mutual support—qualities that are essential, regardless of gender.

Listening to their experiences helped me understand that vulnerability is a universal human trait. It does not diminish one's strength; rather, it enhances our ability to connect with others and navigate life's challenges. This realization inspired me to embrace my own vulnerability more fully, paving the way for deeper connections with those around me.

The Courage to Share

Sharing my fears and uncertainties became an act of courage. I learned that opening up about my diagnosis and treatment allowed others to feel safe doing the same. This collective vulnerability fostered a deeper sense of community among patients, reinforcing the idea that we are all in this together. It became evident that strength is not merely about enduring hardship in silence; it is about fostering connections and supporting one another through the ups and downs of life.

The Broader Impact

Challenging the traditional notions of masculinity extends beyond the individual. As more men share their experiences with breast cancer and embrace vulnerability, we begin to create a cultural shift. This shift can inspire future generations to redefine what it means to be strong and to understand that emotional expression is not just acceptable—it is essential.

A New Definition of Masculinity

Reflecting on my journey, I recognize that the path through breast cancer has fundamentally reshaped my understanding of masculinity. I have come to appreciate that true strength lies in vulnerability and emotional honesty. By sharing my story and challenging societal norms, I hope to contribute to a culture that embraces authenticity—one that values emotional expression and connection across all gender identities.

As we redefine masculinity and vulnerability, we pave the way for a more compassionate society. Together, we can create an environment where everyone, regardless of gender, feels empowered to share their struggles and seek support. In this shared journey, we find strength—not just in our battles against cancer, but in our shared humanity.

Embracing Intersectionality

As I navigated my journey through breast cancer, I also became increasingly aware of the intersectionality of identity—how race, sexuality, socioeconomic status, and other factors play a significant role in the experiences of those facing cancer. This awareness further challenged my understanding of strength and masculinity, prompting me to consider how societal expectations vary across different groups.

Diverse Experiences in the Waiting Room

In the waiting rooms, I encountered individuals from various backgrounds. Each person brought their own narrative, shaped by their unique experiences. For some men of colour, the added layers of cultural expectations and stigmas surrounding health could make expressing vulnerability even more difficult. They faced not only the challenges of illness but also the burden of societal pressure to conform to rigid ideals of masculinity.

Hearing these stories opened my eyes to the broader implications of cancer as a health crisis. It became clear that the fight against cancer is not just a personal battle; it is also a collective struggle that encompasses diverse experiences and challenges. Understanding this intersectionality enriched my perspective and highlighted the importance of creating inclusive spaces where all voices are heard and valued.

Fostering Emotional Literacy

One of the key components of redefining masculinity lies in fostering emotional literacy among men. Emotional literacy refers to the ability to recognize, understand, and express emotions effectively. Many men are raised with the belief that expressing emotions is a sign of weakness, leading to a cycle of emotional repression.

The Role of Humour

Amidst the gravity of our experiences, humour emerged as a powerful coping mechanism. Laughter became a shared language among my fellow patients, providing relief from the stress and anxiety that accompanied our diagnoses. It served as a reminder that vulnerability doesn't have to be sombre; in fact, it can be liberating to laugh at our circumstances, allowing us to reclaim our narratives. By embracing humour, we fostered a culture where it was okay to be both strong and vulnerable—a balance essential for emotional well-being.

Empowering Future Generations

By sharing my experiences, I hope to inspire future generations to approach vulnerability as a strength rather than a weakness. The next generation of men should feel empowered to express their emotions, seek support, and redefine what it means to be masculine in a way that encompasses compassion, empathy, and authenticity. It is vital for young boys and men to understand that their worth is not solely determined by their ability to hide their feelings or bear burdens alone, but rather by their willingness to engage with their emotions and connect deeply with others.

This chapter of my life has been about more than just facing a diagnosis; it has been about challenging societal norms and paving the way for a more inclusive understanding of strength. As I navigated my journey through breast cancer, I encountered numerous individuals who defied traditional expectations of masculinity. Their openness and vulnerability inspired me, reinforcing the idea that sharing our struggles can be profoundly liberating. It is through these shared experiences that we cultivate an environment where emotional honesty is not only accepted but celebrated. The importance of this shift cannot be overstated. When we encourage young men to embrace their emotions, we are not only enriching their personal lives but also fostering healthier relationships and communities. Teaching future generations that it is okay to be vulnerable will help dismantle the stigma surrounding mental health, leading to a society where seeking help is seen as a courageous act rather than a sign of weakness. This change can lead to stronger interpersonal connections and a greater sense of belonging, where everyone feels safe to express their true selves without fear of judgment.

Furthermore, we have the opportunity to engage in conversations that challenge outdated stereotypes of masculinity. By sharing stories—whether they be about joy, grief, love, or fear—we can create a tapestry of experiences that reflects the rich complexity of human existence. This not only helps to humanize the experience of vulnerability but also cultivates a greater sense of empathy among individuals. As we engage in these dialogues, we can encourage young men to stand up against toxic masculinity, creating advocates for change who will foster environments of understanding and support.

Together, we can create a culture where vulnerability is embraced, allowing everyone—regardless of gender—to find strength in their truth. This vision extends beyond just individual growth; it encompasses societal transformation. Imagine a future where emotional intelligence is prioritized alongside academic and professional achievement. In this world, individuals are encouraged to listen, empathize, and collaborate, resulting in communities that thrive on mutual respect and understanding.

Inspiring future generations to redefine masculinity is not merely an individual journey; it is a collective responsibility. By fostering an environment where vulnerability is celebrated, we can empower young people to step into their authentic selves. Let us stand together, advocate for change, and ensure that the next generation understands that true strength is not about being invulnerable but about being open, compassionate, and real. Through this collective effort, we can transform the narrative around masculinity and create a more inclusive, empathetic world for everyone.

Building a Supportive Network

Building a supportive network is crucial, especially during challenging times like facing a serious illness. The importance of having a strong support system cannot be overstated. It serves as a lifeline, offering emotional sustenance, practical help, and a sense of belonging when the world feels isolating. Reflecting on my journey, I realize how vital it would have been to have been guided toward support groups rather than feeling as if I was hanging on the sidelines, grappling with my fears and uncertainties alone.

When confronted with a life-altering diagnosis, such as breast cancer, the initial response can often be one of shock and confusion. It's easy to retreat inward, believing that you need to handle everything on your own. This mindset can lead to feelings of isolation, exacerbating anxiety and depression. I found myself at a crossroads, unsure of where to turn for help or understanding. I wish I had known about the existence of support groups—safe spaces where individuals share their experiences, fears, and triumphs with one another. These groups provide a unique opportunity to connect with others who are on similar journeys, creating a bond that can be incredibly comforting.

Support groups serve several essential functions. First and foremost, they offer emotional support. Sharing your story with others who have faced similar challenges can be cathartic. It normalizes your feelings and helps you realize that you are not alone. Hearing others articulate their fears, frustrations, and victories can validate your own experiences and provide perspective. It creates a space where you can express your emotions freely, without fear of judgment or misunderstanding. This environment fosters a sense of community, where members can uplift each other and remind one another of their inherent strength.

Moreover, support groups often serve as a source of practical information and resources. Members frequently share insights about treatment options, coping strategies, and wellness practices that have worked for them. This collective knowledge can be invaluable as you navigate the complexities of your diagnosis and treatment. I often found myself wishing I had someone to turn to for advice or tips on managing side effects or finding local resources. A support group could have provided that, empowering me to take control of my journey and make informed decisions.

In addition to emotional and practical support, these networks often foster accountability and motivation. When surrounded by individuals who are also striving to navigate their health challenges, there is a natural inclination to encourage one another to take proactive steps. Whether it's attending a doctor's appointment, trying a new wellness practice, or simply getting out of bed on tough days, knowing that others are cheering for you can be incredibly motivating. This sense of accountability can make a significant difference in your overall outlook and willingness to engage with your treatment.

The connections formed in support groups can also extend beyond the meetings themselves. Lifelong friendships can blossom as members bond over shared experiences, providing a deeper layer of support outside the structured group setting. These relationships can be especially meaningful during difficult moments when you might feel like you are losing touch with the world. Having someone who truly understands your journey can make a world of difference, offering a shoulder to lean on when times get tough.

Regrettably, I spent too much time feeling isolated, hanging on the corner of my own emotional landscape instead of reaching out to others. This solitary approach not only prolonged my suffering but also prevented me from experiencing the richness of shared stories and mutual support. If I had been guided to join a support group, I believe my journey would have been marked by greater resilience and less loneliness. It is a stark reminder that reaching out for help is not a sign of weakness; rather, it is a courageous step toward healing.

As I reflect on my experience, I am driven by a desire to advocate for the importance of building supportive networks. I urge others who may find themselves in similar situations to seek out these resources and embrace the power of community. Whether through formal support groups, online forums, or local meetups, there are countless opportunities to connect with others who share your experiences. It's important to remember that you do not have to face your journey alone.

In conclusion, building a supportive network is essential for emotional well-being during difficult times. The strength found in community cannot be overstated. By reaching out, sharing our stories, and supporting one another, we can create a powerful force for healing and resilience. I wish I had had the foresight to join a support group during my own journey; I am confident it would have enriched my experience and provided the connection and understanding I craved. Moving forward, let us prioritize the creation of supportive networks, fostering environments where vulnerability is celebrated and where everyone feels empowered to share their journey. Together, we can navigate life's challenges with strength, compassion, and solidarity.

A New Paradigm of Strength

As I conclude this chapter, I am reminded that strength transcends gender. It is not confined to rigid definitions; rather, it is found in the willingness to be vulnerable, to share our stories, and to support one another through life's challenges. The notion that strength is synonymous with invulnerability is outdated and limiting. True strength is multifaceted and exists in the rich tapestry of human experiences, characterized by our ability to connect deeply with ourselves and others.

By redefining masculinity and embracing the emotional landscape of our experiences, we can foster a more compassionate and understanding society. This redefinition requires us to challenge traditional stereotypes and to recognize that emotions are not weaknesses but integral parts of our humanity. As we embark on this journey, we create spaces where individuals feel empowered to be their authentic selves—allowing for a true celebration of strength in all its forms. This means recognizing that nurturing relationships, showing empathy, and seeking help are not signs of weakness, but hallmarks of a courageous and resilient individual.

In this new paradigm, we must acknowledge the profound impact of sharing our vulnerabilities. When we openly discuss our struggles, we not only lighten our own burdens but also create pathways for others to do the same. This sharing can take many forms— conversations among friends, storytelling in public forums, or even writing about our experiences. Each act of vulnerability contributes to a culture where emotional honesty is valued and where individuals can lean on one another during difficult times. In this shared space, we learn that we are not alone in our struggles and that support can come from the most unexpected places.

As we look forward, let us commit to building a society where the new paradigm of strength is rooted in empathy, vulnerability, and understanding. This shift will require continuous effort and dedication from all of us—men and women alike. It will involve listening to each other's stories, advocating for emotional openness, and championing the idea that vulnerability is not a sign of weakness, but rather a path to greater strength.

Imagine a world where future generations of men and women can navigate their emotional landscapes without fear of judgment or ridicule. A world where expressing feelings, seeking support, and showing compassion are celebrated as strengths. This vision is attainable, and it starts with us embracing and embodying this new paradigm of strength in our everyday lives. Together, we can create a legacy that redefines what it means to be strong, fostering a society where every individual feels valued, understood, and empowered to express their true selves. This commitment to change is not just for ourselves; it is for those who will come after us, ensuring that they inherit a world where strength is defined by our ability to connect and uplift one another in our shared journey of life.

Chapter 6

Reflections on Identity and Transformation

Reckoning with Change

Cancer is an experience that reshapes life in ways you can't fully understand until you've walked that path. The disease itself, and everything that comes with it, becomes more than a physical battle—it's a reckoning with identity, with what you thought you knew about yourself, and with what truly matters. Cancer doesn't care about your gender, your plans, or your carefully constructed image of who you are; it strips you down to your core.

For both men and women, the moment of diagnosis is shattering. In an instant, life splits into a "before" and an "after," and everything that felt solid—the routines, the plans, even the body you thought you knew so well—feels uncertain. But it's in that uncertainty that we're forced to confront a deeper question: *Who are we when everything we've taken for granted is stripped away?*

I had always seen myself through the lens of strength and self-reliance. I took pride in those qualities, believing they were markers of resilience. But cancer made me realize that true resilience comes not from holding tight to old definitions of strength but from allowing myself to change—sometimes painfully, sometimes slowly, but always toward something more real.

Confronting Vulnerability

Facing cancer pushes you into a space of vulnerability that is both frightening and freeing. For so long, I associated vulnerability with weakness. I believed, as many of us are taught, that the strongest people are the ones who can face life's challenges alone, without showing fear or pain. But the truth is, vulnerability isn't weakness—it's humanity.

For men and women alike, there's a societal pressure to uphold certain roles. Women often feel the weight of being caretakers and emotional anchors, while men are expected to be stoic and self-reliant. But illness breaks down those expectations. It forces you to accept help, to admit fear, and to open up about your pain. And in that process, I learned that real strength isn't about enduring silently. It's about allowing yourself to be seen fully—fear, sadness, hope, and all. Cancer put me in a position where I had to depend on others. I had to let people into a part of my life that I normally would have kept private. At first, that felt unnatural, like I was losing control. But gradually, I began to understand that accepting support didn't make me weak; it connected me to the people who truly cared. Vulnerability allowed for deeper relationships, both with myself and others.

Rebuilding Identity

Cancer changes how you see yourself—there's no avoiding that. For me, it altered my physical appearance, and that was difficult to accept at first. The scars from surgeries became visible reminders of what my body had endured. They were marks of survival, yes, but also symbols of loss. I had to grieve not only the physical changes but also the person I used to be before the diagnosis. But through that grieving came the opportunity to rebuild my identity in a way that was truer, more honest. I began to let go of the idea that strength meant perfection or invulnerability. Instead, I embraced the idea that strength comes from adaptability, from being able to face change head-on and still find a way forward. This is a lesson that applies to all of us, regardless of gender: the way we define ourselves isn't static. It's fluid, constantly shaped by our experiences, challenges, and growth.

For women, who often deal with body image pressures and expectations around appearance, the physical toll of cancer can feel particularly heavy. And for men, admitting to feeling vulnerable about their bodies or their emotional state can seem like a betrayal of everything society teaches them about masculinity. But what I have come to realize is that strength and identity don't need to fit into those narrow boxes. Our bodies—scarred or changed—are living proof of endurance. Our willingness to adapt, to shift our sense of self, is the real measure of resilience.

Transformation Through Struggle

There's a cliché we often hear: *what doesn't kill you makes you stronger.* I've found that it's not quite that simple. Struggle transforms you, but the strength you gain isn't always about becoming harder or tougher. Sometimes, it's about becoming softer, more open, and more in tune with the fragility of life.

Cancer forced me—and forces everyone who faces it—to see life differently. It's not about just surviving the illness, but about what you take from the experience. For me, that meant learning to accept that life's greatest challenges often come with the most profound growth. It also meant letting go of outdated ideas of who I should be and embracing who I could become.

This process of transformation doesn't happen all at once. It's slow, painful, and often involves taking steps backward before moving forward. But that's okay. Growth isn't linear. For women and men alike, it means giving ourselves permission to be imperfect, to grieve what's been lost, and to slowly, patiently build something new from the ashes of those losses.

Moving Forward With Purpose

The path forward is about more than survival—it's about living with intention, embracing the new identities we've built in the wake of our struggles. Cancer taught me that life is fragile, and that fragility is a reminder to live more fully, to connect more deeply, and to be more present in the moments that matter. It also taught me that I have a responsibility to share what I've learned—to remind others that they're not alone in their battles and that transformation is possible, even in the darkest times.

For both men and women, moving forward with purpose means acknowledging that our stories don't need to fit into traditional moulds. We don't have to live up to unrealistic expectations of what it means to be strong or successful. Strength is found in showing up, in facing fear, and in choosing to keep moving forward, even when the path ahead is unclear.

In the end, this experience has given me a new sense of purpose—not just for myself but for others, too. I want to be part of a conversation that redefines what it means to be strong, vulnerable, and resilient, regardless of gender. We can all build lives where our struggles become our strength, where our scars—whether physical or emotional—become symbols of our capacity to endure and thrive.

Once you've faced a life-altering challenge like cancer, the idea of "normal" becomes almost laughable. For so long, we chase the notion of returning to how things were—physically, emotionally, mentally. We long to be who we were before the diagnosis. But the reality is, you can't go back. The landscape has changed, and with it, so have you. What I've learned is that the real journey isn't about returning to a past version of yourself, but about embracing the new normal.

The idea of a "new normal" isn't easy to accept, and it takes time to process. At first, it felt like a concession—as if I was admitting defeat. But eventually, I realized that this new normal wasn't a compromise; it was a transformation. Cancer didn't erase who I was—it added new layers, new depth, new meaning to my life. I became more attuned to my body, more aware of my mental and emotional health, and more grateful for the relationships and experiences that bring richness to life.

For men, this can be particularly challenging. We're conditioned to value stability and control, to see change as a threat. But in reality, change is the only constant. Cancer taught me that clinging to the past is a futile effort. Instead, I had to learn to adapt, to be flexible, and to welcome the uncertainty of this new chapter. This isn't just about cancer—it's a lesson we can all carry into any of life's challenges.

For women, the concept of the new normal often intersects with societal pressures around appearance, caregiving, and emotional resilience. The physical and emotional scars of cancer can feel like a betrayal of those expectations, but they can also be a form of liberation. The new normal is an opportunity to shed the weight of those societal pressures and redefine what it means to live fully, authentically, and unapologetically.

A huge part of embracing this new normal is learning to accept yourself—completely and without reservation. It sounds simple, but for most of us, it's anything but. Self-acceptance means coming to terms with the parts of ourselves we might prefer to ignore: our weaknesses, our scars, our fears, and our failures. But it also means recognizing and celebrating our resilience, our strength, and our capacity for growth.
In the early stages of my diagnosis, I struggled with self-acceptance. I felt disconnected from my body, betrayed by it. It was hard to look at myself in the mirror and see someone different from the person I'd been before—someone with scars, someone who had lost parts of themselves, both literally and figuratively. But over time, I realized that those scars were not something to be ashamed of. They were symbols of what I had endured, of the battles I had fought and won. They became a part of my story, and learning to

accept them was a crucial step in healing—not just physically, but emotionally.

Self-acceptance isn't a one-time achievement; it's a practice. It's something we have to work on every day, especially in a society that often places impossible standards on appearance, success, and emotional stoicism. But when we cultivate self-acceptance, we open the door to true freedom. We no longer have to live up to anyone else's expectations. We are free to be who we are, in all our complexity, our beauty, and our imperfections.

Breaking Down Gendered Expectations

One of the most important realizations that came to me during my cancer journey is how deeply ingrained societal expectations about gender are—and how limiting they can be. Men and women are both conditioned to fulfil specific roles, and those roles often leave little room for vulnerability, emotional honesty, or real connection.

For men, the expectation to be strong, stoic, and emotionally self-sufficient can be suffocating. When faced with something like cancer, those expectations can feel impossible to meet. How can you be "strong" in the traditional sense when your body is failing you? How can you be stoic when you're scared for your life? The truth is, those expectations aren't just unrealistic—they're harmful. They isolate men from the support and connection they need during their most vulnerable moments.

For women, the pressures are different but equally restrictive. Women are often expected to be the emotional caregivers, to keep things together even when they're falling apart themselves. When women face serious illness, they can feel a double burden: the need to fight their own battle while still being a source of strength for others. The expectation to remain nurturing and composed in the face of adversity can rob women of the space to truly process their own pain.

Breaking down these gendered expectations is essential—not just for individuals dealing with illness, but for society as a whole. We need to create a culture where men feel comfortable expressing fear, sadness, and vulnerability without shame, and where women feel empowered to put their own needs first without guilt. Strength isn't about fitting into a narrow definition of what it means to be masculine or feminine. Strength is about being fully human, in all our complexity.

Reconnecting with Your Body

One of the most challenging aspects of the cancer experience, for both men and women, is the way it changes your relationship with your body. Before my diagnosis, I took my body for granted. It was something I used, something I pushed to its limits without much thought. But cancer changed all of that. Suddenly, my body was something fragile, something unpredictable. It felt like a stranger.

The process of reconnecting with my body was slow and difficult. At first, I resented the physical changes—the scars, the fatigue, the sense that my body had betrayed me. But over time, I began to see my body not as a source of weakness, but as a vessel of resilience. It had endured the unthinkable. It had fought back. And in that fight, I discovered a newfound respect for it.

For women, the relationship with their bodies can be even more fraught, especially in a culture that places so much emphasis on physical appearance. The changes that come with cancer—whether it's hair loss, weight fluctuations, or surgical scars—can feel like a personal loss. Yet, those changes reflect survival. Reclaiming your body after cancer is not about returning to how things were, but about embracing how things are now, and recognizing the beauty in that transformation.

Reconnecting with your body also means learning to listen to it in a new way. Before cancer, I pushed through pain, ignored fatigue, and treated my body as if it were indestructible. Now, I understand that self-care is not a luxury—it's a necessity. Paying attention to what my body needs, whether it's rest, nourishment, or simply kindness, has become an essential part of my healing process.

One of the most important lessons I've learned through this journey is that healing is not a linear process. There are good days and bad days, moments of strength and moments of despair. Sometimes you feel like you're making progress, and then out of nowhere, you're hit with a wave of grief, fear, or frustration. That's okay. That's normal.

For so long, I believed that healing was something you completed, a destination you eventually arrived at if you worked hard enough. But I've come to understand that healing is more like a journey without a fixed endpoint. It's something that unfolds over time, with setbacks and breakthroughs, moments of clarity and moments of confusion. It's messy, it's unpredictable, and it's ongoing. This realization has been freeing. It's allowed me to be gentler with myself, to accept that I don't have to have it all figured out. I can take things one day at a time, one step at a time. Some days, just getting out of bed is an accomplishment. Other days,

I feel like I'm capable of anything. Both days are valid. Both are part of the process.

As I continue to reflect on my journey, I realize that the version of strength I once held onto was limited. It was based on an idea that strength meant power, control, and invulnerability. But true strength is so much more than that. It's about flexibility, about adapting to change, about finding courage in moments of fear and uncertainty. Strength isn't about standing tall when everything is going right. It's about getting back up when everything has fallen apart. It's about allowing yourself to be vulnerable, to ask for help, and to admit that you're struggling. It's about finding beauty in the broken places and meaning in the pain. For men and women alike, this is the new vision of strength I've come to embrace. It's a strength that transcends gender, that defies traditional roles, and that speaks to the heart of what it means to be human. We are all stronger than we think, not because we can endure without breaking, but because we can break and still find a way to heal.

In the end, cancer does not define the entirety of my story. It's a chapter, a defining one, but not the final one. What I've come to understand is that the meaning of this journey isn't found in the diagnosis or the treatments. It's found in how we respond to those moments, in how we choose to move forward. The journey isn't about becoming the person you were before—it's about becoming the person you were always meant to be. It's about discovering new depths of strength, compassion, and resilience within yourself. It's about learning to live with uncertainty, to embrace change, and to find joy

Chapter 7

The Role of Family and Friends

Navigating the Journey with Support and Solitude

As I embarked on my journey with breast cancer, I confronted a harsh truth: I was navigating this battle alone. Though I had friends and acquaintances, the absence of immediate family—those who often provide the support many lean on during difficult times—was keenly felt. My parents no longer existed in my life, and the familial connections I once had were fraught and distant, lacking the nurturing support typically expected. However, this chapter isn't solely about my solitude; it serves as a reflection on the diverse roles that friends and family play in the lives of those facing illness. Some choose to stand steadfastly by our side, while others may withdraw out of fear or uncertainty. Still, some linger in the background, remaining distant figures in the shadows. Each of these dynamics illuminates the intricate tapestry of human relationships, revealing how they shape our experiences during times of adversity.

The Dichotomy of Support

For many, the presence of family and friends becomes a cornerstone of strength and resilience during a health crisis. Their unwavering support can transform a daunting journey into one shared with love and encouragement. However, I also witnessed how fear can drive people away. Friends sometimes vanish when confronted with the reality of illness, grappling with their own fears of vulnerability or the misconception that they might "catch" the disease. This behaviour can be heartbreaking for those battling illness. It reminds us that not everyone has the emotional capacity to confront their own fears, let alone support someone else through theirs. It's essential to recognize that this reaction is not a reflection of the person fighting the illness but rather the complexities of human emotion and fear. Conversely, I've seen how profound and uplifting it can be to have beautiful friends and family by your side. Their presence becomes a beacon of hope and strength, illuminating even the darkest days. These individuals remind us that we are not alone in our struggles. They laugh with us, cry with us, and most importantly, they listen without judgment.

For those fortunate enough to have such support, the journey becomes not just about surviving but also about thriving amid adversity. Each shared moment, every word of encouragement, builds a fortress of emotional resilience that can help withstand the toughest challenges. These connections become lifelines, allowing us to navigate our experiences with greater hope and determination. Yet, for many who find themselves in solitude, it's easy to feel forgotten and overwhelmed. To those who feel abandoned, I want to extend a message of hope: You are not alone.

Even when it feels like darkness surrounds you, know that there is light within you. The journey may be solitary, but that does not diminish your strength or your ability to fight.

Reflecting on my own experiences, I found that even in solitude, I could cultivate a relationship with myself—a bond that became essential for my mental and emotional well-being. I learned to reach deep within for resilience, to express my fears through journaling, and to seek solace in small joys, like a favourite book or a quiet moment in nature. In my loneliness, I discovered the power of self-compassion, which helped me face each day with renewed strength. To those who have family and friends, I encourage you to cherish that support. Engage in open conversations about fears, expectations, and the realities of illness. Your loved ones might be grappling with their own emotions, and discussing these can foster understanding and closeness.

For those who feel abandoned, consider reaching out in whatever ways you can. There are communities, both online and in-person, filled with individuals who understand your journey. Seek connections where you can find understanding and camaraderie among those who have walked similar paths.

Finally, let's acknowledge those who may not have anyone at all. There is beauty in the human spirit's capacity to endure, and even when surrounded by silence, your story matters. Your journey is uniquely yours, filled with lessons that can inspire others. Know that there is hope, even in loneliness, and that your strength can shine brightly despite the challenges you face.

As I reflect on my journey, I hold in my heart the complexities of human connection. The presence of friends and family can be a blessing, while their absence can be a profound lesson in resilience. Whether surrounded by loved ones or facing the journey alone, there is strength to be found. May we all strive to build bridges of understanding and compassion, ensuring that no one has to walk their path in silence.

When we confront our struggles—whether through personal reflection, writing, or online forums—we create spaces that, while not directly shared, resonate with others facing similar challenges. This act of vulnerability can be incredibly healing. In my own journey, I found that acknowledging my fears, frustrations, and hopes alleviated some of the burdens I carried. In a world where silence often prevails in the face of adversity, speaking out becomes a revolutionary act. It serves as a reminder that we are not defined solely by our struggles but also by our resilience. By recognizing these narratives, we foster an unspoken bond of solidarity that transcends physical distance, allowing us to feel connected even in solitude.

Support groups can be invaluable in this journey, providing a structured space where individuals can connect over shared experiences. These groups offer a platform for exchanging stories, receiving advice, and finding solace among those who understand the complexities of illness. For those who find it difficult to access in-person support, online communities have blossomed, creating virtual havens for sharing, learning, and healing. In these spaces, friendships can form across geographical boundaries, proving that connection is possible even when physical presence is not.

While my own journey was marked by solitude, I discovered that isolation could also be a teacher. It forced me to turn inward, to ask myself difficult questions about my desires, fears, and the meaning of resilience. This introspection helped me cultivate a deeper understanding of my own strength, transforming solitude into an opportunity for growth. Many who feel isolated may initially view their circumstances as a weakness, but it's crucial to recognize the potential for personal empowerment that exists in these moments. Embracing solitude can lead to self-discovery and foster a sense of independence that is invaluable, not just in facing illness but in all areas of life.

As I reflect on the various ways friends and family can influence our experiences, I recognize the importance of compassion—not just towards ourselves but also towards those who may not know how to provide support. Sometimes, friends and family may withdraw due to their own discomfort with illness or their inability to navigate their feelings. Understanding this dynamic allows us to foster compassion for those around us, recognizing that their actions stem from fear or confusion rather than a lack of love or care. This perspective can ease the heartache of abandonment, helping us find peace in our circumstances.

If you find yourself in a situation where friends have distanced themselves or family is absent, consider actively seeking new connections. Engage with community resources such as local support groups, workshops, or online forums that resonate with your journey. Often, the people we meet in these settings become not just allies in our struggles, but also friends who uplift and inspire us. Building these new relationships takes courage, especially when vulnerability feels risky. However, the rewards can be profound. New friends often provide fresh perspectives and can serve as reminders that community is always within reach, even if it must be actively sought out.

One of the most profound realizations I've had is that everyone has their own battles to fight, often hidden beneath the surface. While I was grappling with my health, I began to see the pain and struggles in others—friends, acquaintances, and even strangers. This awareness deepened my empathy, reminding me that no one is immune to hardship.

At times, I felt hurt and abandoned by the absence of support from those I hoped would be there for me. However, upon reflection, I recognized that this distance might stem from their own fears and uncertainties. Many people may not know how to navigate the complexities of someone else's diagnosis, and their hesitation can often act as a defence mechanism. Understanding this allowed me to approach the situation with compassion, leading to deeper reflections on vulnerability and the struggles we all face in our own ways.

Beyond emotional support, family and friends play a critical role in managing the practicalities of daily life during a cancer journey. Treatment can be exhausting, making even routine tasks feel daunting. Loved ones can step in to assist with daily chores, meal preparation, and errands, alleviating some of the burdens that accompany illness. This practical help not only eases the physical strain but also allows the patient to focus on healing. Additionally, having someone accompany the patient to medical appointments can be invaluable. This companionship provides emotional reassurance and helps ensure that important questions are raised, and medical information is accurately understood. Friends and family can also assist in managing healthcare needs, such as organizing medications and keeping track of symptoms.

Maintaining social connections is another crucial aspect of support during a cancer journey. Friends and family can help the patient stay connected to their social circles by organizing gatherings or simple check-ins that provide a sense of normalcy and community. Engaging in enjoyable activities together—whether watching movies, sharing meals, or participating in hobbies—creates moments of joy that serve as vital distractions from the weight of illness. Celebrating milestones, whether completing a round of treatment or achieving personal goals, also plays an essential role in fostering a sense of accomplishment and joy. Acknowledging these victories reinforces the idea that hope and resilience are very much alive, even in the face of adversity.

In the unfortunate event of loss, family and friends become essential in navigating the complexities of grief. Their shared experiences provide invaluable support in processing emotions and finding a path toward healing. The presence of loved ones serves as a poignant reminder that even in the darkest moments, no one has to face their struggles alone.

Finding Strength Together

Supporting someone through cancer is a complex reality. It demands emotional fortitude, patience, and an understanding that no words can fully ease the pain. As I supported several people with different forms of cancer, I realized that the gift of presence—simply being there when it matters most—can be a lifeline. In those moments of hardship, I learned that true friendship is defined by unwavering support and compassion. Through these experiences, I witnessed firsthand the power of resilience and the strength drawn from genuine connection.

Caregivers can come from any walk of life—family members, friends, partners, neighbours, or even compassionate volunteers. Their role in a cancer journey is not confined by a specific title or relationship; anyone who offers support, whether practical, emotional, or both, is a caregiver. Caregivers are often the silent backbone, providing stability and comfort, and their contribution extends far beyond simple tasks. The role of a caregiver is limitless in its scope. It can range from helping with daily chores, attending medical appointments, managing medications, and offering a comforting presence, to being a source of emotional support during the most vulnerable moments. Caregivers often offer companionship during times of isolation and help the patient maintain a sense of normalcy amidst the chaos of illness. Their impact is profound—whether they're providing meals, lending an ear, or simply holding a hand during a difficult procedure, caregivers offer strength when it's needed most. The role requires flexibility, patience, and compassion, as the needs of the patient can change daily. At times, caregivers act as advocates, ensuring the patient's voice is heard in medical settings, while also being a grounding presence in the everyday moments.

In essence, caregivers are indispensable, and their contributions cannot be overstated. Their role is boundless, as they are often called upon to wear many hats—nurse, emotional anchor, organizer, and friend. Whether someone offers support for a day or over the course of an entire treatment, their presence has a lasting, immeasurable impact.

Chapter 8

Life After Cancer

Emerging from the shadow of cancer treatment is a transformative experience, marked by a blend of relief, gratitude, and uncertainty. For many survivors, the journey doesn't end with the last treatment; rather, it opens a new chapter in life—a chapter that invites exploration, adaptation, and personal growth. In this chapter, I reflect on my own experience of finding a new normal after cancer, sharing the challenges and triumphs that shaped my path forward.

The initial relief I felt upon completing treatment was overwhelming. I had fought hard, endured surgeries, and navigated a whirlwind of emotions. Yet, as I settled back into my life, I quickly realized that the victory was only part of the story. The real challenge lay in redefining my sense of self and learning to embrace the changes that cancer had wrought in my life. In those first few weeks, I was often caught off guard by how I felt. Some days, I'd wake up with a sense of purpose, eager to embrace the world and all its possibilities. On other days, a cloud of doubt and fear would loom over me, making it hard to see beyond the scars—both physical and emotional. I learned that this ebb and flow of feelings was normal; recovery is not a straight line but rather a series of ups and downs that require patience and self-compassion.

Finding a new normal meant re-evaluating my daily routines. I discovered that activities I once took for granted, such as going for a run or spending hours on my feet, required careful consideration and adaptation. Instead of pushing through pain or fatigue, I learned to listen to my body. Gentle yoga became my ally, offering a way to move while honouring my limits. I found solace in nature, taking walks that allowed me to connect with my surroundings and ground myself in the present moment.

As I navigated these changes, I also sought to deepen my understanding of health and wellness. I became more mindful of what I put into my body, exploring nutrition that supported my recovery and boosted my energy. Cooking became a joyful exploration; I experimented with fresh ingredients and wholesome recipes, transforming my kitchen into a space of creativity and healing. This shift not only nourished my body but also revitalized my spirit, reminding me that I could take an active role in my health.

Emotionally, I embarked on a journey of self-discovery. I began journaling, allowing my thoughts and feelings to flow onto the page. It became a powerful outlet for processing my experiences, fears, and hopes. Through writing, I uncovered layers of my identity that had been overshadowed by cancer. I realized that my experience did not define me; rather, it was a part of my story—a chapter that I could integrate into the larger narrative of my life.

As I continued to move forward, I found myself daring to dream again. I began to envision a life brimming with new possibilities, one where I could finally pursue passions I had once set aside. Driven by my enduring curiosity for the human mind, I enrolled in online psychology courses, reigniting my love for understanding both myself and others. Though the path to discovering my new normal was fraught with challenges, it was equally rich in moments of triumph. I learned to celebrate the small victories—whether it was rising from bed without pain, savouring a meal with friends, or completing a long-abandoned project. Each accomplishment deepened my resilience and fuelled my determination to keep moving forward, no matter the obstacles. Ultimately, emerging from cancer treatment was not about returning to who I was before; it was about becoming someone new— someone more attuned to the fragility and beauty of life. I discovered that while I might bear the scars of my journey, they were also symbols of survival and transformation. My experience taught me that moving forward is not just a destination but an ongoing process of growth and self-discovery.

As I continue to navigate this new chapter, I carry with me the lessons learned, the relationships forged, and the understanding that life is an ever-evolving journey. In embracing the uncertainties and possibilities ahead, I find hope and excitement for what lies beyond. The end of treatment often brings a rush of emotions. After months of doctor visits, infusions, and side effects, the prospect of "finished" can feel exhilarating yet daunting. For me, the moment I received the news that my treatment was complete was bittersweet. As I celebrated the end of a difficult chapter, I also confronted the uncertainty of what lay ahead. I didn't have to undergo chemotherapy or radiotherapy, treatments many cancer patients face. While this brought a sense of relief and gratitude, it also left me feeling somewhat isolated in my experience. Even without those treatments, my recovery was still full of challenges. The impact of surgery on my body and spirit was profound, shaping my healing in a deeply personal way. My scars became constant reminders of what I had survived—symbols of pain, strength, and resilience. I often traced them with my fingers, feeling a mix of vulnerability and pride in everything they represented.

In the immediate aftermath of my treatment, I experienced a profound sense of disorientation. The routine that had once defined my life—a cycle of appointments, treatments, and follow-ups—was suddenly absent. I found myself standing at a crossroads, uncertain about how to move forward. The adrenaline that had carried me through treatment began to fade, leaving space for a different kind of reality to settle in. As I attempted to reclaim my life, I quickly realized that recovery wasn't just about physical healing; it was a multifaceted process involving emotional, mental, and spiritual dimensions. The fatigue that lingered was not merely a result of my surgery but also an echo of the emotional weight I had been carrying. I felt as if I was navigating a fog, unsure of what lay ahead.

Finding balance in this new reality required patience and self-compassion. I had to learn how to take things one day at a time, allowing myself to feel whatever emotions arose without judgment. I began to practice mindfulness, which helped ground me in the present moment. It became a tool to navigate the chaos swirling in my mind, reminding me to breathe deeply and acknowledge my feelings as they came. Each deep breath was a gentle reminder that I was alive and capable of moving forward, even when the path felt unclear.

As I gradually shifted my focus to recovery, I also began to reassess my priorities and values. What truly mattered in my life? I found myself drawn to activities that nourished my soul and provided solace. I began to explore creative outlets, picking up a paintbrush for the first time in years. The act of creating became therapeutic; it allowed me to express emotions that I couldn't always articulate with words. With each stroke of colour on the canvas, I felt a sense of release, as if I were reclaiming pieces of myself that had been lost in the whirlwind of treatment. Additionally, I explored creative writing, experimenting with poetry and short stories. Each piece became an exploration of my emotions, a way to express what I couldn't always articulate in conversation. I wrote about resilience, hope, and the complexity of my feelings as a cancer survivor. Through this creative process, I began to see my experience not just as a series of challenges but as a source of inspiration and strength.

The journey of recovery was not without its setbacks. There were days when I felt overwhelmed by the sheer weight of my experiences. I grappled with feelings of survivor's guilt, questioning why I had been spared the harsher treatments that many of my peers endured. Yet, through these moments of doubt, I found strength in the understanding that every survivor's story is valid, regardless of the specifics of their treatment. As I began to find my footing, I also embraced the notion of redefining what "normal" meant for me. I realized that my life would never return to what it once was, and that was okay. In fact, it presented an opportunity for growth and exploration. I began to set new goals, not just in terms of health but also in my personal life. I sought to reconnect with friends, rekindling relationships that had been strained during my treatment. I travelled to places I had long wanted to visit, embracing life with an open heart and a sense of adventure.

Emerging from treatment, I understood that this new chapter was one of exploration and self-discovery. I was determined to embrace every moment and to live fully and authentically. Each day became an opportunity to celebrate small victories and acknowledge the progress I was making. In reflecting on this transition, I recognized that while the journey from treatment to recovery is deeply personal, it is also a shared experience that connects us to one another. The path may be fraught with challenges, but it is illuminated by moments of joy, resilience, and growth. I emerged from the shadow of treatment not just as a survivor, but as a person ready to embrace life with renewed purpose and gratitude. The aftermath of surgery was more than just a physical recovery; it required a complete revaluation of my capabilities. Fatigue lingered like an unwelcome guest, forcing me to navigate a new normal regarding my energy levels and physical abilities. Each day felt like a negotiation between what I wanted to accomplish and what my body was ready to handle. I quickly learned that healing is a process, and recovery does not follow a linear path. There were days when I felt strong enough to tackle the world, only to be met with unexpected waves of exhaustion that left me resting more than I had anticipated.

The side effects of treatment, while different from those experienced by individuals undergoing chemotherapy or radiotherapy, persisted in their own ways. I had to contend with pain, both physical and emotional, as I processed the events that had unfolded. It required patience and self-compassion to recognize that healing wouldn't happen overnight. I often had to remind myself that it was okay to take things slowly, to honour my body's signals, and to prioritize rest. Emotionally, I was navigating a complex landscape. The relief of finishing treatment was accompanied by anxiety about recurrence. Questions about my health loomed over me like a dark cloud: Would the cancer come back? How could I ensure I was living fully after such a profound experience? These fears were palpable, but they were matched by an unexpected sense of freedom.

I realized that adjusting to life after cancer would require intentional effort and self-discovery. I had been given a second chance—a rare gift that many long for. Yet, with that gift came a responsibility to explore what it meant for me to live fully. I found myself grappling with questions about my identity and purpose in this new chapter. Who did I want to be now, and how could I honour the journey that had brought me to this point? Embracing this opportunity meant stepping outside of my comfort zone and engaging with the world in ways I had previously overlooked. I began to seek out experiences that ignited my passion and inspired me to connect with others. Whether it was diving into new hobbies, volunteering in my community, or simply savouring moments of joy in everyday life, I was determined to make the most of my newfound perspective. This journey of self-exploration required me to confront fears and insecurities, but it also opened doors to unexpected possibilities. I learned that living fully wasn't just about grand gestures; it was about finding beauty in the ordinary, cherishing relationships, and cultivating gratitude for the small things that often go unnoticed. With each step I took, I embraced the complexity of this journey, understanding that it was not merely about survival but about thriving in a world that felt both familiar and profoundly different.

However, while I embraced this newfound perspective, I soon discovered that the road ahead was not without its obstacles. The financial toll of my cancer treatment became a significant hurdle I had not fully anticipated. With the inability to work during my treatment, I lost a crucial source of income, leaving me struggling to support myself. Once treatment ended, I found it difficult to re-enter the job market. Many positions required a level of physical stamina and focus that I wasn't sure I could provide, and the prospect of interviews felt daunting. As I grappled with everyday living expenses—rent, groceries, and utilities—I found myself in a precarious situation. Covering these basic needs felt overwhelming, and I turned to debt as a temporary lifeline. I began searching for ways to "find money," relying on loans, credit cards, and borrowing from friends. Each decision, while necessary, added weight to the financial burden I carried.

The struggle to manage my finances left me feeling trapped. Just when I thought I had turned a corner in my recovery, the stress of mounting debts cast a shadow over my progress. I lay awake at night, anxiety gnawing at me as I wondered how I would navigate this new reality while also focusing on my health. Each new expense felt like a reminder of my limitations, and I wrestled with guilt and frustration. I knew that prioritizing my health had been essential, but the pressure to regain financial control was immense. While the road ahead remained challenging, I was committed to navigating both my physical and financial recovery. Each small victory in managing my finances provided a renewed sense of empowerment and hope for the future, reminding me that even amid struggles, there were still opportunities for growth and stability.

Back in 2017, I felt utterly alone in my struggle, unaware of the myriad support associations and networks available to cancer survivors. I grappled with both my health and financial burdens, feeling lost without guidance on where to turn.

In my darkest moments, I often felt isolated, as if the challenges I faced were unique to me. I had not been informed about local organizations or community programs that could have provided assistance, whether it was emotional support, financial guidance, or career resources. The absence of this information deepened my sense of hopelessness. I wished I had known that others were out there— people who had walked similar paths and found their way through the fog. When I finally discovered these associations years later, it was as if a light had been turned on in a dark room. Learning about their existence was both a relief and a source of frustration; I had needed their help when I was at my most vulnerable, yet no one had pointed me in their direction. Organizations focused on cancer recovery offered workshops, financial counselling, and peer support groups that could have alleviated some of my struggles much earlier in my journey. I realized that this wealth of information had not been available to me during my treatment. Only in the years following my recovery did I come across these resources, particularly with the rise of worldwide cancer awareness initiatives, like October Rose in France. This month-long campaign has not only heightened awareness of breast cancer but has also fostered a global community of support for those affected by the disease. As stories of survival and strength flooded social media and public events, I began to see how interconnected we all are in this fight. The surge in visibility has led to increased funding for research, improved patient resources, and a broader conversation about the importance of mental and emotional well-being in cancer care. It became clear that these initiatives were vital in shaping a more informed and supportive environment for survivors like myself, who once navigated their journeys in relative isolation.

Years after my surgery, I visited several physiotherapists who were shocked to learn that I had never been prescribed physiotherapy to address my post-surgery issues. This oversight had resulted in chronic pain and discomfort that I still grapple with today. It became clear that, while awareness was growing and information was becoming more accessible, I had navigated my challenges in isolation, unaware of the support that could have lightened my burden. These encounters with healthcare professionals highlighted not only the gaps in my own care but also the importance of comprehensive support systems for cancer survivors. The physiotherapists offered insights and tools that could have significantly improved my recovery and quality of life, reminding me that my journey didn't have to be solitary.

Reflecting on this, I became passionate about raising awareness of the support systems available to cancer survivors. I wanted to ensure that no one else would have to navigate their recovery feeling abandoned or uninformed. Each step I took toward my recovery served as a reminder of the importance of community and the power of shared experiences. It was a bittersweet realization—knowing that I could have benefited from this support back in 2017—but it fuelled my determination to advocate for others who might be in similar situations. it becomes clear that everyone's path is unique yet interconnected through shared experiences. For those battling cancer, the journey is often a complex interplay of emotions, where embracing healing requires acknowledging the challenges that arise. What does it mean to face these hurdles while remaining open to the possibility of recovery? It's essential to explore the resources available, as many may exist just beyond the horizon, waiting to offer support during the most vulnerable times.

For caregivers supporting loved ones through cancer, the role played in their journey can be both profound and transformative. Consider the ways in which emotional encouragement can complement practical assistance. Listening, sharing fears, and celebrating even the smallest victories can forge a bond that strengthens both the caregiver and the one in treatment.

And for those grappling with fear surrounding illness—whether contemplating the "what ifs" or witnessing someone they love struggle—transforming that fear into empowerment is crucial. Educating oneself about cancer, not merely as a daunting disease but as a journey many have navigated, can illuminate the path through uncertainty. This understanding fosters compassion, allowing for a more profound connection to those who are affected.

In a world where the shadows of illness often loom large, it's vital to recognize the light found in connection, understanding, and shared experiences. Each question pondered and every conversation initiated has the power to deepen awareness and reinforce resolve. Together, this collective effort creates a network of support and resilience, uplifting not only the individuals directly impacted but also those who stand beside them.

As the journey continues, the importance of advocating for awareness and support systems for cancer survivors resonates deeply. There is a role for everyone in this intricate dance of healing, and the belief that hope can flourish amidst adversity serves as a guiding light. While the road may be fraught with challenges, it is equally rich with opportunities for growth, connection, and renewal.

Personally, I took the time to envision what I wanted my future to look like, setting both personal and professional goals. These aspirations included pursuing further education and embarking on travel adventures. I also made a conscious effort to prioritize meaningful relationships and experiences. This vision became a guiding star, reminding me that while my past was shaped by cancer, my future could be crafted with intention and purpose. I learned to embrace change and uncertainty, recognizing that life's unpredictability can lead to beautiful opportunities.

Chapter 9

A Tribute to the Women Who Fight Every Day

The journey through breast cancer has illuminated the remarkable resilience and courage of the women I encountered along the way. Each of their stories stands as a testament to the profound strength that emerges in the face of adversity, showcasing not only the battles they fought but the hope they inspired in others. From those who shared their experiences in support groups to strangers in waiting rooms, each woman left an indelible mark on my heart. These women navigated their challenges with grace, facing uncertainty while embodying an unwavering spirit that was contagious. Some were in the thick of treatment, grappling with side effects and the weight of their diagnoses, yet still found the strength to uplift those around them. Others, having emerged from their battles, became pillars of strength, sharing wisdom and encouragement that resonated deeply.

In this chapter, I dedicate my words to these incredible fighters, each one a beacon of hope and resilience. Their stories are linked in a rich collage of shared experiences, reminding us all of the power of community and solidarity. It's a celebration of their unwavering spirit and the powerful impact they have had on my life and the lives of countless others. Together, they create a chorus of strength that echoes far beyond their individual struggles, illuminating the path for those who follow.

Through their journeys, I have learned that vulnerability can coexist with strength, and that sharing our stories can forge connections that heal. The impact of their courage extends beyond mere survival; it instils a sense of purpose and belonging in a world that often feels overwhelming. In honouring them, I am reminded that our collective voices can inspire change and foster understanding in ways we may never fully comprehend. Each day, I carry their stories with me, committed to honouring their legacy by advocating for awareness, support, and the celebration of life itself.

The Strength of Women

Throughout my life, I have been continually amazed by the strength of women, a force that often surpasses that of men in both resilience and grace. This strength manifests in various forms—emotional, physical, and spiritual—shaping not only their lives but also the lives of those around them. Women embody a remarkable blend of courage, empathy, and tenacity that enables them to face numerous battles, often with a beauty and dignity that leave an indelible mark on the world.

From my mother to my friends and even acquaintances, I have witnessed firsthand the extraordinary power women possess in navigating life's challenges. My mother, for example, faced hardships with a quiet strength that often concealed her struggles. She balanced the demands of raising a family and working tirelessly, all while managing her own fears and uncertainties. Her ability to transform adversity into valuable lessons of perseverance showcased her resilience. Although the emotional and physical toll of her personal battles was significant— and truly deserving of an entire book to explore—she remained a steadfast pillar of support for those around her. Her journey demonstrated that true strength is often rooted in selflessness and love.

Similarly, my friends have shown me that strength is not just about enduring challenges but also about supporting one another in times of need. I have seen women come together, forming a network of solidarity that provides comfort and encouragement. In moments of despair, they uplift each other with shared laughter and tears, creating a safe space where vulnerabilities can be expressed without fear of judgment. This interconnectedness amplifies their strength, reminding us all that we are not alone in our struggles.

Acquaintances I have encountered have also shared their own narratives of resilience. Whether battling illness, overcoming personal loss, or navigating societal pressures, these women often rise above their circumstances with remarkable courage. They fight not just for themselves but for their families, communities, and the next generation. Their strength serves as a reminder that the fight against adversity is not merely an individual struggle but a collective effort that resonates through time and space.

Despite their incredible strength, I often wish these women didn't have to face such numerous battles. Life can be an unforgiving arena where women must continuously prove their worth, often in the face of systemic challenges. Whether it's dealing with health issues, societal expectations, or the weight of caregiving, the burdens can be heavy. Yet, even in the darkest moments, they manage to rise, illuminating the path for others who may feel lost.

Their battles are not just evidence of their strength; they also reflect a broader narrative about the challenges women face in society. The relentless fight against stereotypes, discrimination, and inequities can be exhausting. Yet, in confronting these battles, women forge identities steeped in resilience and empowerment. Their ability to transform pain into purpose creates a powerful legacy, inspiring others to challenge their limitations and strive for their own dreams.

In celebrating the strength of women, I am reminded that beauty and power coexist in a delicate balance. Women possess an innate ability to be both fierce and nurturing, strong and vulnerable. It is this duality that enriches their experiences and the lives of those they touch. They redefine what it means to be strong—not as an absence of fear or pain but as the courage to face those emotions head-on. The power of women transcends individual narratives; it creates a collective force capable of transforming the world. Each woman's journey, characterized by distinct challenges and triumphs, contributes to a more extensive foundation of resilience. By sharing these stories, we not only honour their struggles but also empower future generations to recognize and harness their own capabilities. This remarkable force is multifaceted, deserving of our acknowledgment and celebration. It inspires us to recognize our resilience, support one another, and work toward a future where the challenges women face are fewer and less overwhelming. Let us commit to amplifying their voices, ensuring that their courage is celebrated and deeply ingrained in the essence of our society.

Courage in Vulnerability

After my own journey through cancer, I encountered many female friends who are also battling the disease, some still fighting as I write this. Through their experiences, I have come to understand the profound strength that can be found in vulnerability. These remarkable women openly share their fears, pain, and the uncertainties that come with their diagnoses. This openness fosters a space for authenticity, allowing us to connect on a deeply human level. I have witnessed firsthand the courage it takes to expose oneself emotionally, sharing not only polished narratives of strength but also the raw, unfiltered realities of their struggles. In supporting one another, we cultivated an environment where vulnerability became a source of empowerment. Women who may have once felt isolated in their struggles found comfort in knowing their experiences resonated with others.

Perseverance Through Trials

The perseverance displayed by these remarkable women was not merely a response to the challenges they faced—it became the essence of their journey. From the first moment of diagnosis, they were thrust into a world of uncertainty, where every day presented new battles to be fought. The path ahead was often steep, marked by a relentless series of treatments and invasive procedures that tested both their bodies and spirits. Yet, despite the physical pain and emotional strain, they continued to press forward with a determination that was nothing short of extraordinary.

What struck me most was not just their resilience in the face of treatment but their ability to maintain a sense of grace through the darkest moments. Each day brought new uncertainties: Would the next round of chemotherapy bring relief or more suffering? Would their bodies withstand the next surgery? How would they reconcile the fear of recurrence that seemed to linger even on the good days? These questions weighed heavily on their minds, yet they never allowed them to define their existence. Instead, they chose to focus on the moments of joy that punctuated their struggle—small victories, a shared laugh, or even the quiet strength found in simply enduring another day.

In many ways, their perseverance was not just about survival; it was about reclaiming agency in a situation where so much felt beyond their control. They made choices, however small, that reaffirmed their strength and willpower. Whether it was showing up for treatment with a smile, supporting a fellow patient, or refusing to let fear dictate their lives, these women found ways to assert their power, even in the face of adversity.

As I witnessed their journeys unfold, I realized that perseverance is not a singular act of courage but a continuous process of choosing to move forward, even when the road seems endless. It's the decision to keep fighting when hope feels distant, to confront fear with unwavering resolve, and to rise each morning with the determination to make it through another day. These women redefined what it meant to be resilient—not as an absence of fear or hardship, but as the relentless pursuit of life in all its complexity, beauty, and struggle. Their perseverance also extended beyond their personal battles. Many of these women became advocates for others, using their own experiences to raise awareness and build communities of support. They shared their stories, offered guidance, and stood as beacons of hope for those just beginning their journey. In doing so, they transformed their pain into purpose, ensuring that their trials were not endured in vain but served as a source of strength for others facing similar paths. It is through these acts of perseverance, both seen and unseen, that the true strength of these women shines brightest. Their ability to endure and rise above their challenges serves as a powerful reminder of the boundless capacity of the human spirit. In their stories, we find not only inspiration but also the courage to face our own trials with a little more hope, a little more grace, and a lot more determination.

Witnessing a woman's journey toward accepting her body after cancer has been one of the most profound and eye-opening experiences of my life. As an observer, I was reminded time and again of the complexity of that relationship women have with their bodies, one that's often shaped by societal expectations, personal identity, and, in many cases, the pressures of femininity. Watching someone close to me, whether it a dear friend or an acquaintance, go through this journey gave me a new perspective on the deep emotional layers involved in body acceptance— something that extends far beyond physical appearance.

For many women I've known, the struggle to accept a body altered by cancer wasn't just about coping with scars or physical changes—it was about redefining their sense of self. Losing a breast, losing hair, or gaining scars after surgery and treatment can feel like losing a part of who they are, especially in a world that often ties a woman's worth to her physical appearance.

It was heartbreaking to see the women I loved questioning their beauty, femininity, or identity because of these changes. Yet, at the same time, it was incredibly inspiring to witness the strength it took for them to come to terms with those feelings.

As a man, I could only witness this journey from the outside, but that vantage point allowed me to appreciate how intense and powerful the relationship between women and their bodies can be. The women I saw fighting for body acceptance weren't just battling physical changes, but also the internalized expectations of what their bodies were "supposed" to represent. For many, this meant redefining what it meant to be feminine or beautiful—realizing that these concepts weren't tied to having perfect hair, smooth skin, or unblemished features. Instead, beauty became about resilience, survival, and a deeper, more meaningful connection with their bodies.

One of the most powerful realizations for me was that body acceptance doesn't follow a straight line—it ebbs and flows. There were moments when I saw these women embrace their bodies with confidence, only to struggle again on more difficult days. It reminded me that acceptance isn't about reaching a state of perfection; it's about showing up every day, despite the pain or discomfort, and choosing to see one's body as worthy and valuable, just as it is. I've learned that for many women, accepting a body altered by illness is a deeply personal and ongoing journey. It requires immense courage, not only to face the physical changes but also to confront the emotional weight that comes with them.

I will forever admire the women I've witnessed on this path—their bravery in the face of uncertainty, their ability to keep moving forward even when it feels impossible, and their determination to find beauty and meaning in their bodies, regardless of scars or changes. Witnessing this acceptance has left a lasting impact on me, reminding me of the profound strength it takes to embrace vulnerability, redefine beauty, and love oneself in a world that doesn't always make that easy. These women have taught me that true beauty lies in resilience, and that the journey of acceptance—whether of the body, mind, or soul—is one of the most courageous acts a person can undertake. The importance of speaking up and breaking free from isolation cannot be overstated, especially in times of illness or hardship.

Having experienced both silence and the impact of shared stories, I've come to realize how vital it is to reach out, be vulnerable, and connect with others. Whether it's a cancer diagnosis, personal loss, or another life-altering event, there's often a tendency to retreat, either out of fear of burdening others, shame, or the belief that no one else could understand the depth of your struggle. However, silence can become a heavy burden. Bottling up emotions and attempting to manage fear, pain, and uncertainty alone can intensify feelings of loneliness. I've witnessed this in people I love and felt it myself during difficult moments. The idea of staying quiet, as though it could shield us from the harshness of our reality, only deepens the sense of isolation, making it harder to find clarity or healing.

One of the greatest lessons I've learned is that sharing your struggles—whether with close friends, family, or others—isn't just helpful; it's necessary. Opening up creates space for understanding, empathy, and support. By speaking out, we allow others to share in the journey, offering comfort and reminding us that we are not alone. This act of sharing is healing, not just for the person expressing their feelings but for those listening, too. Hearing someone else's story can reveal that our fears, doubts, and pain are not unique, breaking the illusion of being isolated in our experiences.

I recall when a close friend began to open up about her fears. For a long time, she carried herself with immense strength, but beneath that exterior was a vulnerability she had kept hidden. When she finally spoke about her anxieties, frustrations, and moments of despair, it was as though a weight had been lifted. It not only helped her process her emotions but also brought us closer. Late-night conversations filled with tears and laughter showed me that these moments of connection were just as important to her healing as any medical treatment.

Talking doesn't just relieve emotional pressure; it creates a sense of community. It invites others to share their stories and offer support, fostering solidarity. When we open up, we often realize that others have walked similar paths, and this can be profoundly reassuring. It reminds us that others have endured and survived, and that we, too, can navigate the darkness. For those facing illness, trauma, or loss, this shared connection is invaluable. In contrast, isolation magnifies helplessness. By cutting ourselves off, we lose the opportunity for perspective, support, and resources that could make the journey easier. Isolation can erode the spirit, deepening sadness into depression and creating a dangerous cycle of withdrawal. But when you choose to speak up, you break that cycle. You create opportunities for new connections—whether through a support group, finding someone with a similar experience, or simply being heard after a long period of silence. These moments can spark hope, even in the darkest times. Ultimately, speaking up isn't just about releasing emotions—it's about forging meaningful bonds that remind us of our shared humanity. It's about recognizing that fear, pain, and uncertainty are universal experiences. By voicing them, we allow others to step forward with compassion and understanding, breaking down the walls of isolation and building pathways toward healing. We are reminded that, no matter how difficult the journey, we don't have to face it alone.

Acknowledging the Unseen Battles

Behind every smile, every handshake, and every casual greeting, there often lies a world of unseen battles that most of us fail to notice. These battles are fought quietly, away from public view, often without recognition or praise. They can take many forms— physical illness, mental health struggles, financial hardship, or emotional trauma—but they share one common thread: the profound courage required to face them every day. It's easy to assume that the strongest people we know are those who appear unfazed by life's challenges. We admire their resilience, their calm under pressure, and their ability to navigate difficulties without showing cracks in their armour. But the truth is, strength doesn't always look like confidence. It often looks like vulnerability, exhaustion, or quiet perseverance. Strength, in many cases, is simply the act of showing up—of continuing to face the day despite the weight of invisible struggles pressing down.

In the context of illness, for instance, the physical battle is the one that's most readily acknowledged. We can see the effects of chemotherapy, the toll of surgeries, the visible signs of a body in pain. But what about the internal battles, the mental and emotional struggles that accompany illness? The fear that gnaws at you when you're lying awake at night, the anxiety that accompanies every doctor's visit, the constant negotiation between hope and despair—these are the battles that often remain hidden. And yet, they are just as real, just as draining, and sometimes even more difficult to face than the physical ones.

Having witnessed these struggles firsthand, especially in women who have battled cancer, I've come to realize how essential it is to acknowledge these unseen battles. This idea extends beyond illness. Many people fight daily battles that go unnoticed by those around them. Take, for instance, the person dealing with depression, who musters every ounce of energy just to get out of bed in the morning. Or the single parent juggling multiple jobs to make ends meet, constantly battling exhaustion and financial stress while trying to create a stable life for their children. Or the individual grappling with grief after the loss of a loved one, struggling to find their way through a world that suddenly feels foreign and empty. These battles are often unseen because they don't manifest in ways that are immediately visible to others. But they are battles nonetheless, and they require just as much courage and strength as the ones we can see.

For women especially, the unseen battles are compounded by societal expectations. Women are often expected to be caregivers, to be emotionally available, and to maintain their composure even in the face of immense personal hardship. This can create an added layer of pressure, as many women feel the need to suppress their struggles in order to meet these expectations. They may hesitate to speak openly about their pain or exhaustion, fearing judgment or the perception that they are not "strong enough." But this only adds to the burden they carry.

Acknowledging these unseen battles requires us to look beyond the surface. It requires empathy, the willingness to understand that everyone is carrying something, even if it's not immediately apparent. It means creating spaces where people feel safe to share their struggles without fear of judgment. It means recognizing that the quiet endurance of hardship is a form of strength, even if it doesn't fit the conventional image of resilience.

One of the most powerful ways to acknowledge these unseen battles is through conversation. Talking about what we're going through—whether it's physical illness, mental health challenges, or emotional pain—can help to break down the barriers of isolation. When we speak about our struggles, we invite others to do the same, creating a culture of openness and support. This can be particularly important for those whose battles are less visible, as it gives them permission to voice their pain and to seek help without feeling ashamed or weak.

At the same time, we must learn to listen—to really listen. So often, people give subtle hints about what they're going through, hoping that someone will pick up on their unspoken needs. By listening with empathy and attention, we can better understand the weight of the burdens others are carrying, and we can offer support in meaningful ways. Sometimes, the simple act of being present—of offering a kind word, a gesture of support, or even just a listening ear—can make all the difference.

It's also important to remember that acknowledging unseen battles doesn't mean trying to fix them. Many struggles have no quick fix, and it can be frustrating for those going through them when well-meaning friends or family try to offer solutions instead of support. Sometimes, what people need most is validation—an acknowledgment that what they are going through is hard, that their pain is real, and that they are not alone. This kind of acknowledgment can be incredibly healing in and of itself.

Ultimately, acknowledging the unseen battles of those around us is about practicing empathy and compassion. It's about understanding that everyone's journey is unique, and that the struggles we can't see are often the ones that require the most courage. It's about creating a culture where vulnerability is not seen as a weakness but as a natural part of the human experience. By doing so, we can help to lift some of the burden off the shoulders of those who are fighting these unseen battles, offering them the support and understanding they need to continue their journey with strength and hope.

Mental Health and Healing

The mental toll of cancer can be profound, often overshadowing the physical challenges that accompany the disease. Many individuals grapple with feelings of anxiety, depression, and isolation long after treatment has ended. While medical professionals typically focus on addressing the physical aspects of cancer, the emotional and psychological strain can be overwhelming, lingering long after the immediate threat has passed. For many women, this mental burden becomes a quieter battle, fought in the solitude of their thoughts.

Anxiety, depression, and isolation are common experiences that can arise at various points along the recovery journey. Even when the body begins to heal, the mind can remain trapped in fear, uncertainty, and emotional exhaustion. Every ache or pain can reignite the anxiety that cancer might return, while the weight of what has been endured can lead to a feeling of emotional drain. Months or even years of battling the disease, enduring surgeries, treatments, and relentless uncertainty can create a profound sense of mental fatigue. Unlike physical wounds, which can be seen and treated, the emotional scars of cancer often go unnoticed or unaddressed.

Beyond the diagnosis itself, the aftermath can lead to emotional dissonance. On one hand, there's relief and gratitude for having survived; on the other, there is an undeniable grief for the life that once was. The body, once a source of confidence and identity, may now bear scars or changes that affect self-esteem and self-perception. This shift in self-image can significantly impact mental health, leading to a persistent feeling of loss or inadequacy. Depression often emerges as women grapple with what feels like a stolen version of themselves, trying to reconcile the physical and emotional transformations they've undergone.

Furthermore, the support systems that rallied during treatment often begin to wane once the most visible aspects of the cancer journey—chemotherapy, radiation, and surgeries—come to an end. The isolation that creeps in after treatment can become one of the most challenging aspects of recovery. Friends and family, though well-meaning, may believe that the worst is behind them, often overlooking the emotional and psychological healing that still requires attention. Women are left to navigate these turbulent emotions alone as the outward markers of illness fade, and the world expects them to return to "normal." This isolation deepens the mental strain, making it increasingly difficult to voice feelings of fear or sadness when everyone around them celebrates their survival.

For many, therapy, counselling, or peer support groups become essential lifelines. The ability to talk openly about fears of recurrence, the emotional exhaustion that accompanies treatment, and the uncertainty of the future is vital. Acknowledging these emotions can serve as a powerful form of healing. Understanding that others have walked similar paths and experienced the same fears helps to alleviate the feelings of loneliness that often accompany recovery. It becomes a reaffirmation that their struggles are valid and that mental health deserves as much care and attention as physical healing.

Recognizing mental health as a crucial component of cancer recovery is an act of self-compassion. For women who have faced cancer, healing is not solely about surviving the disease; it is about granting themselves permission to feel, to grieve, to express their pain, and to seek help. Mental health must be viewed as an integral part of the recovery process rather than an afterthought. To heal fully, the emotional toll must be recognized, addressed, and embraced as a vital part of the journey toward wellness.

Ultimately, understanding the profound mental impact of cancer encourages us all—whether survivors, caregivers, or medical professionals—to create environments where women feel safe to express their true emotions without fear of judgment or the pressure to remain perpetually strong. By prioritizing mental health, we honour the full spectrum of what it means to heal, acknowledging that the road to recovery encompasses not only the restoration of the body but also the nurturing of the mind and soul.

A Celebration of Courage

I pay tribute to the extraordinary women who bravely fight every day—those whose resilience serves as a guiding light, inspiring and uplifting others while paving the way in their darkest moments. Each story shared is not just a narrative of survival; it embodies the profound power of courage and perseverance. These women remind us that even in our most challenging times, we are never truly alone. As we celebrate these remarkable women, we are called to carry their spirit with us in our daily lives. Their journeys, marked by both hardship and triumph, invite us to embrace the fullness of our own experiences. We honour their legacy by choosing to live with intention, cherishing each moment, and fostering a sense of gratitude that transcends our individual struggles. Their strength becomes a source of inspiration, encouraging us to navigate the complexities of life beyond cancer with courage and determination.

The impact of these women extends far beyond their personal battles. By sharing their stories and openly discussing their vulnerabilities, they challenge societal norms around illness, strength, and femininity. They remind us that vulnerability is not a weakness but a powerful expression of authenticity that fosters connection and solidarity. In a world that often demands unyielding strength, they teach us the importance of embracing our emotions, seeking support, and recognizing that it is okay to lean on others.

Let us not only honour their courage but also amplify their voices, ensuring that their legacies endure in the hearts of those they have touched. It is our collective responsibility to support one another, create safe spaces for dialogue, and challenge the stigma surrounding mental health and the emotional toll of illness. By doing so, we pave the way for future generations, empowering them to face their challenges with the same tenacity and grace that these women have exhibited.

In celebrating their courage, we also acknowledge the strength within ourselves. Each of us has the capacity to be advocates for change, to uplift others, and to contribute to a community that prioritizes empathy and understanding. Let us honour the legacies of these remarkable women by committing to a future where no one feels isolated in their battles and where the collective strength of our shared experiences illuminates the path for those still on their journey.

As we move forward, may the stories of these incredible women resonate within us, guiding our actions and inspiring us to cultivate hope and resilience in our own lives. Together, we can transform our shared experiences into a powerful beacon of light, illuminating the way for those who come after us. In doing so, we ensure that their courage is not just celebrated but continues to inspire and uplift, creating a lasting impact on the lives of all who encounter their stories.

Chapter 10

Breaking the Stigma

Raising Awareness for Male Breast Cancer

When I was diagnosed with breast cancer, the first question I often encountered was, "But isn't that a women's disease?" This reaction, while not uncommon, laid bare a widespread and deeply ingrained misconception about breast cancer in men. It highlighted a profound stigma surrounding male breast cancer—one that can silence voices, diminish experiences, and prevent men from seeking the help they desperately need. This stigma feeds into a larger narrative that breast cancer is exclusively a women's issue, ignoring the reality that men, too, are affected by this potentially life-threatening disease.

Male breast cancer does exist, yet it remains shrouded in a cloak of misconception and misunderstanding. The reality is that, while it is rare—accounting for about 1% of all breast cancer cases—it is very real, and its existence should not be diminished or overlooked. Each diagnosis represents a man who faces not only a significant health challenge but also societal perceptions that can undermine his experience, often making the journey through illness more isolating and emotionally taxing.

For many men, the diagnosis is accompanied by a sense of disbelief—not just from others but often from themselves. Breast cancer, long associated with femininity, forces men into an uncomfortable confrontation with their own vulnerability, challenging ingrained ideas about masculinity. This can prevent men from seeking early medical intervention, potentially worsening outcomes. The unfamiliarity with male breast cancer also means that awareness campaigns, resources, and even medical advice are often geared toward women, leaving men to navigate their diagnoses in uncharted waters.

Further complicating matters is the emotional toll of being diagnosed with a disease that society does not associate with your gender. Men with breast cancer may feel alienated, like they don't belong to the broader cancer community, which is predominantly focused on female patients. This sense of exclusion can intensify feelings of shame or embarrassment, leading some men to remain silent about their diagnosis, thereby reinforcing the stigma. Without visible role models or open conversations about male breast cancer, the cycle of misunderstanding and silence perpetuates itself. It is critical to acknowledge and challenge these stigmas. Awareness and education are key in breaking down the barriers that men with breast cancer face. By openly discussing male breast cancer and highlighting the stories of men who have experienced it, we can begin to change the narrative. Early detection, proper treatment, and emotional support should not be hindered by outdated gender stereotypes. Every individual's experience, regardless of gender, is valid and deserving of recognition.

Ultimately, breast cancer does not recognize gender—it is a disease that affects people, regardless of whether they are male or female. Like any illness, it does not discriminate, and no one is immune from its reach. We must collectively work to dismantle the stigma, so no one feels silenced or sidelined by their diagnosis. Every man and woman affected by breast cancer deserves the same level of care, support, and respect as they navigate this difficult journey.

Challenging Stereotypes

Challenging stereotypes around masculinity and illness is crucial in changing the way society views male breast cancer. The rigid expectations placed on men—often characterized by strength, stoicism, and invulnerability—pose significant barriers to seeking help and openly discussing a breast cancer diagnosis. These societal constructs, which depict men as being impervious to weakness, can make it particularly challenging for male patients to confront and accept their illness, let alone share their diagnosis with others. The stereotype that breast cancer is exclusively a "woman's disease" further intensifies the difficulty. In a culture where masculinity is often equated with physical strength and emotional resilience, admitting to a diagnosis that is typically associated with femininity can feel emasculating. The fear of being perceived as vulnerable or weak looms large for many men, and this can lead to hesitation or outright refusal to acknowledge their illness. In many cases, men might delay seeking medical advice for symptoms they do not associate with themselves, missing early intervention opportunities that could save their lives.

During my own treatment, I was keenly aware of the weight of these societal expectations. The diagnosis was not just a medical challenge but an emotional and psychological one as well. I often found myself grappling with the fear that others might view my illness through the lens of judgment or disbelief. Breast cancer, in many people's minds, was synonymous with women, and my experience with the disease felt almost out of place in that narrative. This sense of isolation, stemming from both internalized and external misconceptions, underscored the need to raise awareness about male breast cancer. It's important to recognize that the perception of breast cancer as a "feminine" disease does more than just perpetuate ignorance—it actively harms men by discouraging them from seeking diagnosis or treatment. For many, acknowledging a vulnerability like cancer conflicts with their deeply ingrained notions of what it means to be a man. This internal conflict can breed feelings of shame and embarrassment, making it even harder for men to discuss their health with others or seek the emotional support they need. The result is an overwhelming sense of isolation, compounded by a society that doesn't acknowledge their existence as part of the breast cancer narrative.

However, breaking these stereotypes is essential for promoting both early detection and proper treatment. By challenging the assumption that breast cancer is gender-specific, we can begin to dismantle the barriers that prevent men from openly discussing their experiences. We need to change the conversation around masculinity and illness, making it clear that vulnerability, far from being a weakness, is a vital part of the human experience. No one should feel less of a man for acknowledging a serious illness, and no one should hesitate to seek care because of societal expectations.

Through my journey, I've come to realize that the act of speaking out—of sharing my story—isn't just about advocating for my own health, but for the health of all men who face similar challenges. Every story shared, every stereotype confronted, takes us one step closer to a world where men feel comfortable acknowledging their illness without fear of judgment. At the same time, it is a tribute to the countless women who have fought and continue to fight breast cancer. Their strength, perseverance, and advocacy have paved the way for all of us, and by sharing my experience, I am standing in solidarity with them. We are all united in this fight, regardless of gender. The more we share, the more we honour the bravery of women and men alike, and together, we move toward greater understanding and support for everyone affected by breast cancer. Raising awareness is not merely a form of advocacy; it's an essential tool for saving lives. By educating others about the realities of male breast cancer, we can ensure that future generations of men feel empowered to take charge of their health, rather than being held hostage by outdated notions of masculinity.

Ultimately, cancer doesn't care about gender. It doesn't discriminate based on societal expectations of who is supposed to be strong or who is supposed to be vulnerable. It's up to us to ensure that these arbitrary stereotypes don't prevent men from accessing the care and support they need. The more we challenge these misconceptions, the more we make space for men to talk about their experiences and take their health seriously. We have the power to change the narrative, to make breast cancer a conversation that includes everyone—not just women, but men too.

Bias in Healthcare

The healthcare system has long operated under the assumption that breast cancer is predominantly a women's disease, which has led to an inadvertent bias toward female patients in diagnosis, treatment, and support. This bias manifests in various ways, often leaving male breast cancer patients underserved, misdiagnosed, or overlooked. One of the key issues is that healthcare professionals, including primary care doctors, oncologists, and nurses, may not be trained or equipped to recognize the early signs of breast cancer in men. Because of its rarity in men—accounting for less than 1% of all breast cancer cases—there is often a lack of awareness among doctors that men can develop the disease at all. This can result in delays in diagnosis as doctors may attribute symptoms such as lumps, swelling, or nipple discharge to more common male conditions like gynecomastia (benign breast tissue enlargement) or infections, rather than considering the possibility of breast cancer. Misdiagnosis or delayed diagnosis significantly impacts prognosis, as early detection is critical for effective treatment.

Moreover, standard medical protocols and guidelines for breast cancer screenings are primarily geared toward women. While women are regularly encouraged to perform self-examinations or undergo mammograms, there are no equivalent guidelines for men, even those who may be at higher risk due to family history. This systemic gap can leave men unaware of potential risks or symptoms, leading to a delay in seeking medical attention. As a result, male breast cancer patients are more likely to be diagnosed at a later stage, when the disease is more advanced and harder to treat.

Healthcare providers also face a steep learning curve when it comes to treating men with breast cancer. Since most treatment regimens and guidelines are based on research conducted on women, men often receive treatment that is tailored to female biology. However, men's bodies respond differently to certain therapies, and side effects may not be the same. For instance, hormone therapy, which is commonly used to treat oestrogen-receptor-positive breast cancer in women, might not have the same efficacy in men or could cause different side effects due to the distinct hormonal makeup in males. There is often a lack of data available to guide healthcare providers on how to adjust these treatments for male patients, forcing them to rely on treatment plans designed for women.

The emotional and psychological support provided by healthcare teams may also fall short for male breast cancer patients. Breast cancer centres, which are typically designed with women in mind, may not have the resources or expertise to address the specific psychological impact of the disease on men. This includes the challenge of confronting societal perceptions of masculinity and the potential stigma of having a disease traditionally associated with women. Men may feel embarrassed or uncomfortable discussing body image issues or sexual health concerns related to their treatment, particularly if their healthcare providers are not accustomed to addressing these issues with male patients.

One of the most significant challenges in treating male breast cancer is the severe lack of research focused on the disease in men. Because male breast cancer is so rare, it has not been a priority in clinical trials or research studies. As a result, the medical community has far less data on the best treatment protocols, prognosis, and survivorship outcomes for men. This gap in research directly affects the quality-of-care male patients receive, as most treatment guidelines are based on studies conducted exclusively on women. For instance, clinical trials on breast cancer therapies often exclude men altogether, meaning that the efficacy and safety of certain treatments for male patients remain largely unknown. Men, therefore, are often treated based on assumptions extrapolated from female-focused studies. However, because male breast tissue is different from female breast tissue in terms of volume, hormone levels, and cell composition, the disease may progress differently in men, and treatments that work well for women may not always have the same impact on men This lack of inclusion in research also means there are few opportunities to explore treatments specifically tailored to men. There could be therapies or interventions that are more effective for male patients, but without male-specific studies, these remain unexplored. For instance, understanding how men metabolize certain drugs differently or respond to chemotherapy could lead to more personalized treatment options, reducing side effects and improving survival rates.

Moreover, the limited research available on male breast cancer makes it difficult for doctors to predict outcomes or provide accurate prognoses for their male patients. Survival statistics and recurrence rates are often derived from female data, which may not fully apply to men. Without more detailed studies on how breast cancer progresses in men, doctors and patients are left with an incomplete picture of the disease, making it harder to tailor follow-up care and long-term survivorship plans.

Another critical area where the lack of research has a profound impact is in understanding the genetic and environmental risk factors for male breast cancer. While it is known that mutations in the BRCA1 and BRCA2 genes increase the risk of breast cancer in men, much remains to be learned about other potential genetic markers or risk factors unique to men. Additionally, the role of lifestyle factors such as diet, alcohol consumption, or exposure to environmental toxins has been widely studied in women but not in men. This limits the ability to offer effective prevention strategies or screening guidelines for men at risk.

To address the bias and research gaps in male breast cancer treatment, the medical community needs to prioritize inclusivity in both clinical practice and research. This means not only raising awareness about male breast cancer among healthcare providers but also ensuring that men are included in breast cancer research and clinical trials. Pharmaceutical companies, research institutions, and cancer organizations must also recognize the importance of studying the disease in men, dedicating resources to better understand how it affects the male population.

Medical guidelines need to evolve to include men, particularly those with genetic predispositions to breast cancer. The development of screening protocols for high-risk men—similar to those that exist for women—would enable earlier detection and better outcomes. Healthcare providers should also be trained to recognize the signs of breast cancer in men and understand the unique challenges they face, from biological differences to psychological impacts. Ultimately, addressing these gaps will not only improve the care men receive but also contribute to a deeper understanding of breast cancer as a whole. By eliminating gender biases and expanding research efforts, we can ensure that all patients, regardless of gender, receive the best possible care.

The Importance of Early Detection and Prevention

When it comes to breast cancer, early detection is critical for increasing the chances of successful treatment and improving survival rates. This is especially true for men, who are often diagnosed at a more advanced stage due to a lack of awareness and screening protocols. While breast cancer in men is rare, accounting for less than 1% of all cases, the importance of recognizing and acting on potential symptoms cannot be overstated. For men, early detection is not only about diagnosing cancer promptly but also about breaking down the stigma that often keeps them from seeking medical advice.

Self-Examination

One of the simplest and most effective tools for early detection is self-examination. Men should regularly examine their chest and breast area, becoming familiar with what is normal for their bodies. Although men may have less breast tissue than women, they can still develop lumps, changes in the nipple, or other symptoms indicative of breast cancer. Conducting a self-exam once a month allows men to detect changes early. Key areas to monitor during self-exams include:

- **Lumps or thickening**: Any new or unusual lump in the chest or underarm area should be considered a red flag.
- **Soreness or pain**: While breast cancer lumps are often painless, any persistent pain in the breast or chest area should be evaluated.

- **Nipple changes**: Look for changes in the nipple, such as inversion, puckering, or discharge, particularly if it is bloody.
- **Skin changes**: Watch for any dimpling, redness, or scaling of the skin around the chest area.

Family History and Genetic Testing

For men with a family history of breast cancer—especially those with close relatives (both male and female) who have had the disease—genetic testing may be an important step. Mutations in the BRCA1 and BRCA2 genes are known to significantly increase the risk of breast cancer in men. If these genetic markers are present, doctors may recommend heightened surveillance, including regular clinical breast exams and possibly even mammograms.

Understanding family history is essential in assessing risk levels. Men who know they are at higher risk should be particularly vigilant about performing self-exams and seeking medical advice for any unusual symptoms. For high-risk individuals, healthcare providers may recommend periodic imaging studies like mammography or ultrasound, especially if abnormalities are detected during physical exams.

Clinical Breast Exams

In addition to self-examinations, men should undergo regular clinical breast exams, particularly if they have risk factors like genetic predisposition or a family history of breast cancer. During a clinical exam, a healthcare professional will palpate the chest and breast area, looking for any abnormalities. These exams are generally more thorough than self-exams and can often changes that might go unnoticed.

While routine mammograms are not standard for men, those at higher risk may benefit from tailored screening protocols under the guidance of a healthcare provider. Many men dismiss potential symptoms, mistakenly assuming that breast cancer cannot affect them. This often leads to delays in seeking medical advice until the disease has progressed, complicating treatment and reducing survival rates.

Overcoming Stigma and Barriers

One of the significant barriers to early detection in men is the stigma surrounding breast cancer. Many men feel embarrassed or uncomfortable discussing changes in their breast area or seeking medical attention for a condition largely associated with women. This cultural stigma can prevent men from taking proactive steps to monitor their health, often leading to delayed diagnoses. Public health campaigns and awareness efforts must evolve to include men in the conversation about breast cancer. Often portrayed as a women's issue, breast cancer awareness campaigns are dominated by pink ribbons and female-centred messaging. While these initiatives have been vital in increasing awareness among women, they can inadvertently exclude men, leading to the misconception that breast cancer is not a concern for them.

Men need to understand that breast cancer is a human disease and, like any illness, it does not discriminate based on gender. Campaigns should encourage men to take control of their health by performing self-exams and openly discussing any concerns with their doctors. By normalizing discussions about male breast cancer, we can reduce the stigma that often prevents men from seeking the early care that could save their lives.

Prevention and Vigilance Are Key

While there are currently no universal screening guidelines for male breast cancer, that does not diminish the importance of vigilance. Self-examination, awareness of family history, and early reporting of symptoms like lumps or discharge are crucial steps that men can take to protect their health. Men should be encouraged to monitor their breast health and engage with healthcare providers when something seems off.

As more men share their stories and awareness increases, the hope is that early detection will become more common among male breast cancer patients. Just as women have been empowered to take control of their breast health, men, too, should feel empowered to protect themselves through early detection and prevention. By raising awareness and challenging the stigma, we can ensure that all individuals, regardless of gender, are proactive in managing their breast cancer risk.

Preventive Measures and Healthy Lifestyle Choices

Preventive measures, particularly in the form of healthy lifestyle choices, play an essential role in reducing the risk of developing breast cancer. Although lifestyle modifications alone cannot guarantee prevention, they can significantly impact overall health and potentially lower the risk of breast cancer. For men, in particular, adopting healthy habits becomes crucial, as breast cancer often goes undiagnosed until later stages. Below, we explore how different lifestyle factors and risk management strategies contribute to reducing the likelihood of developing breast cancer.

Adopting a Healthy Lifestyle

Maintaining a healthy lifestyle is one of the most proactive steps men can take to reduce their cancer risk. This approach encompasses diet, physical activity, and the avoidance of harmful substances, each of which can positively affect health and potentially reduce the risk of breast cancer.

Diet and Nutrition

A well-balanced diet can play a key role in promoting breast health. A diet rich in whole grains, fruits, vegetables, lean proteins, and healthy fats provides essential nutrients that support the immune system and overall well-being. Some studies have indicated that diets high in plant-based foods, particularly those containing antioxidants, may lower the risk of developing cancer by reducing inflammation and oxidative stress in the body.

For example:

- **Cruciferous vegetables** like broccoli, cauliflower, and Brussels sprouts are known for their cancer-fighting compounds.
- **Fatty fish** such as salmon and mackerel contain omega-3 fatty acids, which have anti-inflammatory properties.
- **Whole grains** provide fibre, which can aid in maintaining a healthy weight and improving metabolic health.

Conversely, diets high in processed foods, refined sugars, and unhealthy fats have been linked to an increased risk of various cancers. Processed meats and excessive red meat consumption have been associated with an elevated cancer risk due to the carcinogens created during cooking at high temperatures.

Exercise and Physical Activity

Regular exercise is crucial not only for maintaining a healthy weight but also for reducing the risk of various cancers, including breast cancer. Engaging in moderate to vigorous physical activity has been shown to help regulate hormone levels, particularly oestrogen, which plays a role in breast cancer development in men. Physical activity also reduces insulin resistance and chronic inflammation, both of which are risk factors for cancer. Regular exercise not only improves physical health but also contributes to mental well-being, helping individuals manage stress—a known contributor to overall disease risk.

Limiting Alcohol and Avoiding Tobacco

Excessive alcohol consumption has been directly linked to an increased risk of breast cancer in men. Alcohol can elevate oestrogen levels and damage DNA, both of which contribute to cancer development. Completely abstaining from alcohol or significantly reducing intake may further reduce cancer risk. Tobacco use, while more commonly linked to lung cancer, is a major risk factor for several types of cancer, including breast cancer. Smoking exposes the body to carcinogens that damage cells and contribute to cancerous mutations. Quitting smoking is one of the most effective ways to reduce cancer risk across the board and significantly improve overall health.

Managing Risk Factors

In addition to lifestyle choices, managing specific risk factors is crucial for reducing the risk of breast cancer. Certain factors, such as obesity, hormone treatments, radiation exposure, and liver conditions, increase oestrogen levels in men, which in turn increases the likelihood of developing breast cancer.

Obesity

Obesity is a major risk factor for breast cancer in both men and women. Excess fat tissue increases oestrogen production, and elevated oestrogen levels have been linked to breast cancer development. Men who are overweight or obese also tend to have higher levels of insulin, which can contribute to cancer progression by promoting the growth of abnormal cells.

Maintaining a healthy weight through a balanced diet and regular exercise is essential in mitigating this risk. Men should aim for a body mass index (BMI) within the healthy range and focus on reducing abdominal fat, which is particularly linked to hormonal imbalances.

Hormone Treatments

Men who undergo hormone treatments, particularly those involving testosterone replacement therapy (TRT) or oestrogen-related medications, may face an elevated risk of breast cancer. While TRT is prescribed to treat low testosterone levels, it can sometimes be converted into oestrogen in the body, increasing breast cancer risk. It is important for men undergoing hormone treatments to consult with their healthcare providers about their risk of breast cancer and to be monitored for any early signs or symptoms. Alternative treatments may be available for those at high risk.

Radiation Exposure

Men who have undergone radiation therapy, especially to the chest area, may have an increased risk of developing breast cancer later in life. Radiation exposure can damage the DNA in cells, leading to mutations that can eventually result in cancer. Men who have been treated for conditions like Hodgkin's lymphoma or other cancers involving chest radiation should discuss their breast cancer risk with their doctors and may require more regular monitoring or screening for early detection.

Liver Conditions

Liver diseases such as cirrhosis can impact hormone levels, increasing oestrogen levels in men. Since the liver plays a key role in regulating hormones, liver dysfunction can lead to a hormonal imbalance that increases breast cancer risk. Men with liver conditions should work with their healthcare providers to manage the disease and its effects on hormone regulation.

Encouraging Open Conversations

Dealing with cancer is not just a personal battle; it's a journey that affects everyone around you. Whether you are the one undergoing treatment or a caregiver supporting someone you love, the importance of open communication cannot be overstated. Conversations about cancer can be difficult, fraught with emotions, and often filled with uncertainty. Yet, fostering these discussions is essential for emotional well-being, understanding, and ultimately, healing.

When a loved one is diagnosed with cancer, the ripple effects extend far beyond the individual. Family and friends often find themselves in unfamiliar territory, grappling with their own emotions and feelings of helplessness. They may feel unsure about what to say or how to offer support, fearing that their words might either overstep boundaries or come off as dismissive. This uncertainty can create barriers, leading to silence when what's needed is connection.

Create a Safe Space for Dialogue

To encourage open conversations, it's crucial to create a safe environment where everyone feels comfortable expressing their thoughts and feelings. Here are some ways to foster this atmosphere:

Set the Tone: Choose a relaxed setting for discussions—perhaps during a quiet evening at home or over a casual meal. A comfortable environment can help ease tension.

Be Present: Encourage those involved to put aside distractions like phones or television. Giving your full attention shows that you value the conversation and the feelings being shared.

Use Open-Ended Questions: Prompt discussions with questions that invite deeper thoughts, such as "How are you feeling today?" or "What are your biggest concerns?" This encourages dialogue rather than simple yes-or-no answers.

Validate Emotions: It's vital for family and friends to recognize that the emotions surrounding a cancer diagnosis can be complex. Feelings of fear, sadness, anger, and confusion are all normal responses. Encouraging loved ones to share these emotions openly can lead to a sense of relief and solidarity.

Acknowledge Feelings: Encourage family members to share their feelings without judgment. For example, someone might express frustration over feeling powerless; acknowledging that frustration as a valid response can foster understanding.

Share Your Feelings: If you are the one undergoing treatment, sharing your emotions can also help family members feel more connected. Let them know what you're experiencing, both physically and emotionally.

Discuss Practical Concerns Together

In addition to emotional support, discussing practical matters can also help ease stress for both the patient and their loved ones. Here are some topics to consider:

Treatment Plans: Discussing the treatment journey can help demystify the process and bring clarity. Family members may want to know about the treatment schedule, possible side effects, and how they can assist in day-to-day management.

Support Needs: Talk about specific ways loved ones can help, whether that's providing transportation to appointments, preparing meals, or simply being there to listen.

Future Planning: Conversations about the future can be daunting, but discussing hopes, fears, and plans can provide a sense of control and understanding for everyone involved. This might include practical aspects such as finances, or more emotional aspects like aspirations for recovery.

Facilitating Family Discussions

Facilitating family discussions about cancer can be challenging, but it is crucial for ensuring that everyone feels involved and informed. Here are some strategies to help guide these conversations:

Establish Guidelines for Communication

Creating guidelines can help everyone engage respectfully and openly. Here are some suggestions:

Respect Boundaries: Encourage everyone to be mindful of each other's comfort levels. Some may not be ready to discuss certain topics, and that's okay.

No Judgments: Remind everyone that this is a safe space for feelings—no one should feel criticized for their emotional reactions or thoughts.

Be Honest: Encourage honesty in the discussions. It's okay to express discomfort or confusion, as these feelings are part of the journey.

Utilize Resources for Guidance

Sometimes, families may benefit from external support in navigating difficult conversations. Consider these options:

Counselling or Support Groups: Engaging with a professional counsellor or attending support groups can provide invaluable tools for improving communication and emotional health. This can be particularly useful for families struggling to discuss feelings about cancer openly.

Books and Articles: There are numerous resources available that offer guidance on discussing illness and emotional challenges. Sharing these materials with family members can help everyone understand the importance of communication.

Make It a Continuous Conversation

Encouraging open conversations should not be a one-time effort. It's essential to establish a culture of ongoing dialogue where feelings can be expressed freely over time.

Regular Check-Ins: Schedule regular family discussions where everyone can share updates on how they're feeling and any new concerns or questions that have arisen.

Celebrate Small Victories: Whether it's completing a round of treatment or simply having a good day, celebrating small victories together can foster a positive atmosphere and encourage continued openness.

In a time filled with uncertainty and fear, open conversations can serve as a lifeline for those facing cancer and their loved ones. By fostering an environment of trust, validation, and support, families can navigate this challenging journey together. Encouraging dialogue not only strengthens bonds but also ensures that everyone feels heard and understood. As you embark on this journey, remember that you don't have to face it alone; reaching out and connecting with those around you can make all the difference.

Resources and Support

Navigating a diagnosis of breast cancer can be an overwhelming journey, especially for men who often find themselves in an environment where awareness is limited. However, I want you to know that you are not alone, and there are numerous resources and support systems available to help you through this challenging time, no matter where you are in the world.
Global Support and Resources for Men with Breast Cancer

Explore Global Organizations

Many reputable international organizations are dedicated to providing resources and support specifically for individuals facing breast cancer. For instance, the World Health Organization (WHO) and the International Agency for Research on Cancer (IARC) offer guidelines and valuable information that are accessible globally. The Union for International Cancer Control (UICC) is another excellent resource that connects patients with organizations and services across different countries.

Engage with Local Healthcare Providers

Your health is your priority. Don't hesitate to reach out to local healthcare providers who can offer personalized medical advice tailored to your specific circumstances. Family doctors can help guide you through understanding your risks and screening options. Additionally, local hospitals and cancer centres are excellent places to seek specialized care and support.

Connect with Online Support Communities

Sharing your journey can provide not only relief but also valuable insights. Consider joining online platforms like the Male Breast Cancer Coalition, which connects men with similar experiences, or the Cancer Survivors Network, where you can share your story and find camaraderie. Reddit's Cancer Support Forum is another community where you can ask questions, seek advice, and share encouragement.

Utilize International Helplines

Sometimes, all you need is someone to talk to. Many international helplines are available for immediate support, such as LIVESTRONG and Macmillan Cancer Support. Additionally, don't forget about local helplines specific to your country; they can provide timely assistance when you need it most.

Access Trusted Medical Websites

When seeking information, it's essential to rely on credible sources. Websites like the Mayo Clinic, MedlinePlus, and the National Cancer Institute (NCI) offer comprehensive information about breast cancer, including treatment options, support, and patient education materials.

Local Resources Matter

Encourage yourself to explore local resources available in your area. Look for cancer support groups and financial aid programs that can provide additional assistance tailored to your needs.

Embrace Universal Preventive Measures

Empower yourself with knowledge about self-examination and preventive measures. Regular self-examinations can help you notice any changes early, and advocating for your health by asking questions and seeking second opinions can make a significant difference in your care.

Multilingual Resources

If English is not your first language, fear not! Many organizations, such as Cancer Research UK and the American Cancer Society, provide resources in multiple languages, ensuring that everyone has access to crucial information.

Get Involved in Grassroots Awareness Efforts

Lastly, I encourage you to take action in your community. Whether it's starting conversations about male breast cancer or organizing health talks, every effort counts. Together, we can help raise awareness and foster an environment where everyone feels supported.

You are not alone in this journey. By exploring the resources available to you and connecting with others who understand what you're going through, you can find strength and support. Remember, this is not just a fight against cancer; it's a fight for your health and well-being. Take a step forward today, and know that there is a community out there ready to support you every step of the way.

Online Communities and Forums

The rise of digital technology has transformed how individuals connect, offering numerous online resources and communities for cancer patients.

Social Media Platforms: Facebook groups, Instagram accounts, and X hashtags dedicated to male breast cancer provide spaces for sharing experiences, advice, and encouragement.

Dedicated Websites and Forums: Websites like Inspire and Cancer Support Community host forums where patients can ask questions, share stories, and seek advice from others who understand their journey.

Telehealth Support: Many organizations now offer virtual support groups and counselling sessions, making it easier for individuals to access help from the comfort of their homes.

Encouraging Others to Reach Out

I encourage anyone facing a cancer diagnosis, especially male breast cancer, to explore these resources. There is immense power in community, and connecting with others who understand your journey can make a world of difference. Whether through local support groups, national organizations, or online communities, the support you need is available.

As we continue to raise awareness about both male and female breast cancer, let us also champion the importance of these support systems. Together, we can foster a culture of understanding, acceptance, and hope, ensuring that no one feels isolated in their struggle.

By sharing information about these resources, we empower others to seek help, build connections, and find the strength to face their journeys with courage and resilience. Remember, you are not alone—support is just a conversation away.

Practical Advice for Patients and Caregivers

Navigating the journey of cancer—whether as a patient or a caregiver—can feel overwhelming. The emotional, physical, and logistical challenges that arise often require practical strategies to manage the complexities of treatment and support. I will now share essential advice tailored to both patients and caregivers, helping to empower individuals and foster a sense of agency in the face of adversity.

For Patients: Taking Charge of Your Journey

Educate Yourself

Knowledge is one of the most powerful tools you can possess. Understanding your diagnosis, treatment options, and potential side effects can empower you to make informed decisions about your care.

Ask Questions: Don't hesitate to ask your healthcare team questions about your diagnosis, treatment plan, and any uncertainties you have. No question is too small or trivial.

Seek Reliable Information: Use reputable sources such as the American Cancer Society, the Male Breast Cancer Coalition, and healthcare providers to gather information.

Prioritize Communication

Open communication with your healthcare team, family, and friends is crucial. It helps ensure that everyone involved in your care is on the same page.

Keep a Journal: Document your symptoms, questions, and any side effects you experience. This record can help facilitate discussions with your medical team and ensure nothing is overlooked.

Involve Your Support System: Don't hesitate to involve family and friends in discussions about your care. Their support can provide additional perspective and encouragement.

Create a Support Network

Building a support network can make a significant difference in your emotional well-being.

Join Support Groups: Connecting with others who are going through similar experiences can provide comfort and understanding. Whether in-person or online, support groups can foster a sense of community.

Lean on Family and Friends: Don't hesitate to ask for help from loved ones. Whether it's running errands, accompanying you to appointments, or just being there to listen, their support can alleviate some burdens.

Develop a Self-Care Routine

Taking care of your physical and emotional health is paramount during treatment.

Practice Mindfulness and Relaxation: Techniques such as meditation, deep breathing, or yoga can help manage stress and anxiety. Consider incorporating these practices into your daily routine.

Maintain a Balanced Diet: Eating a nutritious diet can support your body during treatment. Focus on whole foods, including fruits, vegetables, lean proteins, and whole grains.

Stay Active: If your doctor approves, gentle exercise can help improve your mood and energy levels. Activities such as walking, stretching, or swimming can be beneficial.

Prepare for Appointments

Being organized and prepared for medical appointments can help you maximize the time spent with your healthcare team.

Bring a Companion: Having someone accompany you can provide emotional support and help you remember important information discussed during the visit.

List Your Questions: Write down your questions and concerns ahead of time. This ensures that you don't forget to address any important topics during the appointment.

Plan for Side Effects

Understanding potential side effects of treatment can help you prepare for and manage them more effectively.

Discuss Side Effects with Your Doctor: Make sure to talk to your healthcare provider about what side effects you might expect and how to manage them.

Create a Side Effect Management Plan: Develop strategies for dealing with common side effects such as fatigue, nausea, or changes in appetite. This might include scheduling rest periods, using ginger for nausea, or experimenting with small, frequent meals.

For Caregivers: Supporting with Compassion and Care

Educate Yourself

As a caregiver, understanding the patient's condition and treatment can help you provide the best support possible.

Learn About the Diagnosis and Treatment: Familiarize yourself with the medical aspects of your loved one's condition, including treatment options and potential side effects.

Attend Appointments: Accompanying the patient to medical appointments can help you gather information and ask questions directly to the healthcare team.

Practice Active Listening

Being a supportive caregiver involves more than just providing practical help; it also means being present and emotionally available.

Create a Safe Space for Communication: Encourage open conversations about feelings, fears, and concerns. Allow your loved one to express themselves without judgment.

Be Patient: Understand that emotions can fluctuate during treatment. Being patient and empathetic can help your loved one feel supported.

Encourage Independence

While it's important to provide support, it's equally important to encourage the patient's independence.

Respect Their Choices: Empower the patient to make decisions about their care and daily activities. This can foster a sense of control during a time when they may feel powerless.

Encourage Participation in Activities: Support your loved one in engaging in activities they enjoy, whether it's reading, gardening, or watching movies. These activities can provide comfort and joy.

Take Care of Yourself

Caregiving can be emotionally and physically demanding. It's essential to prioritize your own well-being.

Recognize Your Limits: Understand that it's okay to set boundaries. You cannot pour from an empty cup; prioritize self-care and rest.

Seek Support for Yourself: Consider joining caregiver support groups or seeking counselling. Sharing your experiences with others who understand can be incredibly beneficial.

Manage Practicalities

Help the patient manage practical aspects of their care to alleviate stress.

Organize Appointments: Keep a calendar of medical appointments, tests, and treatments to ensure nothing is overlooked.

Assist with Daily Tasks: Offer help with household chores, meal preparation, or transportation to appointments. This can relieve some of the patient's burdens.

Be Prepared for Emotional Challenges

Both patients and caregivers may experience emotional ups and downs throughout the journey.

Acknowledge Emotions: Allow space for feelings of frustration, sadness, or anxiety. Validate these emotions and remind your loved one that it's normal to experience a range of feelings.

Encourage Professional Help if Needed: If emotional challenges become overwhelming, suggest seeking support from a mental health professional. Therapy can provide valuable coping strategies and emotional support.

Empowering Each Other

Whether you are the patient or caregiver, navigating the complexities of a cancer diagnosis requires resilience, understanding, and support. By implementing these practical strategies, you can empower yourselves and each other to face the challenges ahead with courage and grace.

Ultimately, the journey through cancer is not one that should be faced alone. By fostering open communication, building a supportive network, and prioritizing self-care, both patients and caregivers can find strength and solace in their shared experiences. Remember, it's not just about surviving the journey; it's about finding moments of joy, connection, and hope along the way.

Moving Forward

As we move forward, it's crucial to remember that our journeys do not end with treatment. Life after cancer is a new chapter, one that brings its own set of challenges and triumphs. Embracing this new normal requires an understanding that healing—both physical and emotional—is an ongoing process.

Encouraging open conversations about survivorship and the continued need for support will help foster a community where everyone feels seen and heard. By continuing to share our experiences, we empower one another to confront the fears that linger even after the medical journey concludes.

A Call to Action

This book is not just a reflection of my journey; it is a call to action for all of us. To patients, caregivers, and advocates: let us continue to share our stories, support one another, and raise awareness about the complexities of breast cancer—especially male breast cancer. Together, we can create a world where no one feels alone in their struggle and where every voice is valued.

Create Spaces for Conversation: Whether through support groups, online forums, or casual gatherings, let's prioritize creating spaces where open dialogue can flourish. By sharing our experiences and insights, we build a network of understanding and empathy.

Support One Another: As we navigate the ups and downs of life, let's commit to being there for one another. Small acts of kindness—checking in on a friend, offering a listening ear, or sharing resources—can make a world of difference.

Advocate for Change: Together, we have the power to advocate for better awareness, funding, and support for male breast cancer. By raising our voices and sharing our stories, we can influence change and create a brighter future for those who will walk this path after us.

A Call for Unity in the Fight Against Cancer

I am compelled to issue a heartfelt call for unity in the ongoing fight against cancer. This battle is not fought by individuals alone; it is a collective struggle that requires our shared strength, compassion, and determination. Together, we can reshape the landscape of cancer care and support, creating a future where no one has to face this journey alone.

The Power of Togetherness

At its core, the fight against cancer transcends gender, age, and background. It touches lives indiscriminately, creating bonds between patients, caregivers, healthcare professionals, and advocates. Each story of resilience, every battle, and every moment of courage contributes to a larger narrative of hope. It is within this tapestry of shared experiences that we find the true essence of togetherness—an unbreakable bond forged through mutual struggles and support. When we unite, we amplify our voices, making a greater impact on awareness, research, and policy. Every action, no matter how small, creates a ripple effect that can lead to profound change. Together, we can break down barriers, challenge misconceptions, and advocate for the resources and care that every cancer patient deserves.

Embracing Diversity in Experience

In our quest for unity, it is crucial to recognize and embrace the diversity of experiences within the cancer community. Each individual's journey is unique, shaped by personal circumstances, backgrounds, and identities. This diversity enriches our collective narrative, offering valuable perspectives that can guide us in our fight. Let us listen to the voices of all those affected by cancer—men and women, young and old, survivors, caregivers, and advocates. By valuing each story, we foster a culture of empathy and understanding, strengthening our collective resolve. Through inclusivity, we ensure that the specific needs of different communities are addressed, and no one is overlooked or marginalized in this battle.

Cultivating Compassionate Support

Unity in the fight against cancer is not just about advocacy and awareness; it is about fostering compassionate support. Each of us holds the power to make a difference in the lives of those impacted by cancer, whether through simple acts of kindness or active engagement in support networks. A comforting word, a listening ear, or a shared moment of understanding can be transformative for someone facing a cancer diagnosis. By cultivating a culture of compassion, we create a safe space for vulnerability and connection, where individuals can express their fears, hopes, and experiences without hesitation.

Building a Legacy of Hope

The fight against cancer is not only about overcoming challenges but also about building a legacy of hope for future generations. By coming together as a united front, we lay the foundation for advancements in research, treatment, and support systems that will benefit those who follow in our footsteps.

Every step we take—whether advocating for funding, participating in clinical trials, or sharing our stories—contributes to a brighter future. Let us inspire the next generation of advocates, encouraging them to carry forward the torch of hope and resilience.

A Future Fuelled by Unity

As we move forward, let us commit ourselves to this shared mission. Our unity in the face of cancer is a powerful force, one that can drive meaningful change. We must continue to raise awareness, advocate for equitable access to care, and build supportive communities that uplift those in need. This call for unity is not a fleeting sentiment but a lasting promise to stand by one another, lift each other up, and fight for a world where every individual affected by cancer receives the love, support, and resources they deserve.

Chapter 11

Thriving Through Treatment

As I navigated the physical challenges of treatment, I compiled a list of practical strategies that helped me cope. Here are some of the techniques that proved most effective:

1. **Create a Routine:** Establishing a daily routine helped provide structure to my days. I prioritized self-care activities, balanced rest with light movement, and set aside time for relaxation.

2. **Stay Active:** Engaging in gentle physical activity, like walking or yoga, not only helped alleviate some treatment-related fatigue but also improved my mood. I found that listening to my body and modifying exercises as needed was essential.

3. **Nutrition Matters:** Focusing on a balanced diet became a cornerstone of my coping strategy. I incorporated nutrient-dense foods, staying hydrated, and experimenting with different recipes to keep meals enjoyable and appealing.

4. **Explore Complementary Therapies:** I explored complementary therapies like acupuncture, aromatherapy, and massage. These practices provided relief from physical discomfort and fostered a sense of relaxation.

5. **Journaling:** Writing down my thoughts and experiences became a powerful outlet. It helped me process my emotions, track my progress, and reflect on moments of gratitude.

6. **Educate Yourself:** Knowledge can empower. I made it a priority to educate myself about my condition and treatment options. Understanding what to expect during each phase of treatment helped reduce anxiety.

7. **Set Boundaries:** I learned the importance of setting boundaries with social commitments. It was okay to say no when I felt overwhelmed or needed time to recharge.

8. **Celebrate Small Victories:** Acknowledging and celebrating small milestones—like completing a round of chemotherapy or managing a difficult symptom—helped reinforce a sense of accomplishment.

Finding Strength in the Journey

Coping with the physical challenges of breast cancer treatment is a complex and ongoing journey. While the path is fraught with obstacles, it is also rich with opportunities for growth and resilience. Through my experiences, I learned that it's essential to prioritize self-care, seek support, and embrace the strategies that resonate with me.

Each step taken in this journey has contributed to my understanding of not just what it means to cope with cancer, but also how to thrive amidst adversity. By sharing my story and the coping strategies I discovered, I hope to empower others facing similar challenges. Together, we can navigate this journey, finding strength and resilience in the shared experience of battling breast cancer.

Embracing Adaptability

One of the most profound lessons I learned throughout my treatment journey was the necessity of adaptability. Cancer treatment is inherently unpredictable, and what works one day may not be effective the next. Embracing a mindset of flexibility allowed me to navigate the physical challenges with greater ease.

Adjusting Expectations

In the face of treatment, I learned to set realistic expectations. There were days when I felt energized and ready to tackle the world, but other days when simply getting out of bed felt like a monumental task. Instead of berating myself for not keeping up with pre-diagnosis levels of productivity, I focused on accepting my new reality. I adopted a mantra of "progress, not perfection," which helped me celebrate the small wins rather than fixate on perceived shortcomings.

I also learned the importance of adjusting my goals. Instead of planning for elaborate outings or demanding physical activities, I focused on simple joys. A walk in the park, a quiet evening with a book, or a cozy movie night became treasured experiences. By recalibrating my expectations, I discovered beauty in the moments that I had previously overlooked.

Listening to My Body

Throughout treatment, I became attuned to the signals my body was sending. I learned to differentiate between fatigue that signalled a need for rest and fatigue that could be alleviated through gentle movement. This awareness was crucial in navigating the physical challenges of treatment.

On days when I felt particularly drained, I allowed myself the freedom to rest without guilt. Conversely, when I felt a surge of energy, I took advantage of it by engaging in light activities, like gardening or stretching. This responsiveness to my body helped me cultivate a healthier relationship with movement and rest, reinforcing the idea that both are essential components of healing.

The Importance of Nutrition and Hydration

Nutrition played a vital role in my treatment journey. I quickly discovered that what I put into my body could significantly affect how I felt physically and emotionally. The chemotherapy-induced nausea made eating difficult, but I knew that maintaining a balanced diet was essential for supporting my immune system and overall well-being.

Nutrient-Dense Choices

I sought guidance from nutritionists who specialized in cancer care. Together, we crafted a plan that focused on nutrient-dense foods—lean proteins, whole grains, fruits, and vegetables. I learned the importance of antioxidants and their potential role in combating the side effects of treatment.

Incorporating smoothies became a favourite strategy. Blending fruits and vegetables into smoothies allowed me to consume a variety of nutrients in a single serving. I experimented with different combinations, adding ingredients like spinach, bananas, and ginger to create tasty and healthy drinks. These became a staple in my diet, offering a quick and nourishing option when I had little appetite.

Staying Hydrated

Hydration also became a priority. I learned that chemotherapy could lead to dehydration, which exacerbated fatigue and discomfort. I made a conscious effort to drink plenty of water throughout the day. To make hydration more enjoyable, I infused water with fruits, herbs, and citrus, creating refreshing and flavourful alternatives.

Finding Comfort in Routine

As my treatment progressed, I found solace in establishing a comforting daily routine. The predictability of certain activities provided a sense of stability amidst the chaos. I discovered that creating rituals around meals, exercise, and relaxation helped anchor me during turbulent times.

Morning Rituals

I started each day with a morning ritual that set a positive tone. This often included gentle stretching or yoga, followed by a nutritious breakfast and a few moments of mindfulness. Engaging in these practices helped me cultivate a sense of intention and purpose, grounding me before facing the challenges of the day.

Evening Wind-Down

In the evenings, I prioritized winding down with calming activities. I found joy in reading, journaling, or listening to soothing music. This time allowed me to reflect on the day and express gratitude for the moments of joy, no matter how small. These rituals became essential in promoting relaxation and enhancing my overall emotional well-being.

Navigating Social Interactions

The physical changes I experienced during treatment also influenced my social interactions. Many of my friends struggled to understand what I was going through, leading to a complex dynamic in my relationships.

Open Communication

I learned the importance of open communication. Instead of retreating into silence, I made a conscious effort to share my feelings and experiences with those closest to me. This transparency helped my loved ones understand my journey and allowed them to offer support in ways that resonated with me.

For example, I shared my challenges with fatigue, explaining that some days I might not have the energy to socialize. This honesty fostered understanding, and many friends became more mindful of my needs. I appreciated those who checked in, sent messages of encouragement, or offered to spend time with me in low-key ways—like watching a movie or simply sitting in silence.

Creating Boundaries

Setting boundaries became another crucial aspect of navigating social interactions. I realized it was okay to decline invitations or request modifications to plans. By communicating my limits, I empowered myself to prioritize self-care without feeling guilty. Those who genuinely cared for me respected my needs and often found creative ways to engage, ensuring I felt included without being overwhelmed.

Seeking Alternative Therapies

In addition to conventional treatments, I explored alternative therapies to complement my care. These modalities provided additional layers of support, helping me cope with physical and emotional challenges.

Acupuncture and Massage

Acupuncture was particularly beneficial in alleviating some of the discomfort associated with chemotherapy. I found that regular sessions helped reduce nausea and promote relaxation. The practice of acupuncture became a cherished part of my self-care routine, providing a sense of control over my body.

Massage therapy also played a vital role. Gentle massages helped relieve tension, promote relaxation, and improve circulation. I sought out therapists who understood the specific needs of cancer patients, ensuring that the treatments were both safe and effective.

Art and Creative Expression

Engaging in creative outlets became a therapeutic escape. I turned to art as a means of self-expression, finding solace in painting and drawing. The act of creating allowed me to channel my emotions into something tangible, offering a form of catharsis that was both healing and empowering.

Writing also emerged as a powerful tool for processing my experiences. Journaling became a safe space for me to explore my thoughts and feelings, giving voice to my struggles and triumphs. Sharing my story through writing not only helped me cope but also fostered a sense of connection with others facing similar journeys.

The Power of Gratitude

Throughout the treatment journey, I discovered the transformative power of gratitude. In the face of adversity, finding moments to express gratitude shifted my perspective. I began to keep a gratitude journal, jotting down small things I appreciated each day—whether it was a sunny afternoon, a kind message from a friend, or a comforting meal.

Practicing gratitude not only uplifted my spirit but also provided a sense of perspective. In recognizing the positives amid the challenges, I found strength and resilience. This practice became a cornerstone of my emotional coping strategy, reinforcing the idea that hope can coexist with hardship.

Embracing the Journey

Coping with the physical challenges of breast cancer treatment is a multifaceted journey that requires patience, resilience, and self-compassion. As I reflect on my experiences, I realize that embracing adaptability, prioritizing self-care, and seeking support from both loved ones and professionals were key to navigating this chapter.

While the path was fraught with obstacles, it was also rich with opportunities for growth, connection, and healing. Through this journey, I have learned that it is possible to find strength in vulnerability and hope amidst uncertainty. By sharing my coping strategies and experiences, I hope to inspire others facing similar challenges, reminding them that they are not alone on this journey. Together, we can navigate the complexities of treatment, discovering resilience and healing along the way.

As I close this chapter of my journey, I'm reminded of the profound lessons gained—resilience, adaptability, and the unwavering strength within us all. No matter our gender, breast cancer brings unique challenges, but the core of the battle remains the same. Cancer doesn't define us; it pushes us to redefine ourselves in the face of adversity.

To every man and woman who has battled breast cancer or stood by a loved one through the fight, your courage embodies the strength of the human spirit. In our darkest moments, we discover our greatest strengths—not by fighting alone, but by leaning on each other, sharing our stories, and lifting one another up.

This battle is not just a personal one; it is part of a collective movement toward a future where breast cancer is no longer a life sentence but a chapter in a life filled with purpose, love, and hope. The scars, whether visible or hidden, are symbols of courage and resilience—of struggles faced, and even when some don't make it through, their strength and spirit continue to inspire us. In every story, we see the enduring power of the human spirit, no matter the outcome. As we continue to raise awareness, let us honour every voice, every journey, and every story—whether male or female. By doing so, we create a powerful, unified front, breaking down the barriers of stigma and silence. Together, we advocate for better treatments, greater understanding, and unwavering support for all who walk this path. This is our legacy—to leave behind not just tales of struggle, but of triumph, love, and unrelenting hope. To those still fighting, to those in remission, and to those who have lost their battles, your stories live on, inspiring the world to never stop searching for a cure, to never stop caring for one another, and to never give up.

Let this be a call to action: continue the fight, raise your voice, and remind the world that breast cancer knows no gender, but neither does the strength to overcome it. Together, we will rise, and together, we will forge a future where breast cancer is no longer a fear but a conquerable foe. The story does not end here; it only grows stronger with every step forward we take.

As I bring this book to a close, I am filled with an overwhelming sense of hope, gratitude, and reflection. The journey we've walked through together—whether through the lens of my own battles or the stories of others—is not just about survival, but about transformation, resilience, and the undeniable strength that resides in each of us. Cancer, in all its forms, is a harrowing test, but it also reveals the courage we never knew we had.

To you, beautiful souls facing breast cancer, regardless of gender, or any challenge that seems insurmountable, know this: you are not alone. You are part of a vast, invisible community of fighters and survivors who understand the depths of your struggle. In the moments when you feel most vulnerable, remember that true courage is not about being fearless; it's about facing your fears, even when they feel overwhelming. Your journey, with all its hardships, is a testament to your strength and determination.

Embrace every small victory, every step forward, and every act of self-care as a triumph. The road may be long and unpredictable, but it is through these challenges that we find our truest selves. You have the power to not only survive but to thrive—to find light in the darkest of days, to rediscover joy, and to emerge from this battle with a new sense of purpose and resilience.

Let this book be a reminder that while the fight against cancer can feel deeply personal, it is also a shared journey. We walk alongside each other, lifting one another up when the weight of our burdens becomes too heavy. Together, we break the silence, challenge the stigmas, and offer support to those who feel lost or alone.

As I close this final chapter, my greatest hope is that you leave these pages with a renewed sense of strength and an unwavering belief in your ability to rise above any challenges or obstacles that come your way. Whatever lies ahead, trust in your resilience to navigate through them. You are a source of inspiration—not only for yourself but for others seeking the courage to keep moving forward. Stand tall, face each day with determination, and let your light shine brightly as a reminder that together, we can overcome any adversity life presents. May your journey, however difficult, lead you to a place of healing, empowerment, and peace. May you discover within yourself the courage not only to endure but to live fully and boldly, knowing you are never alone in your struggles. Whether facing cancer or any other hardship, you are part of a legacy of survivors, warriors, and thrivers. Your story has the power to inspire countless others to keep moving forward, one step at a time.

About the Author

Meet Chris Cooper, a seasoned motivator, mental health advocate, and holistic well-being coach who understands the intricate interplay between nutrition, mental health, exercise, and environment in fostering overall wellness. With a rich background in leading mental health groups, employing Cognitive Behavioural Therapy (CBT) techniques, and recognizing nutrition as a fundamental pillar of well-being, Chris is dedicated to empowering individuals on their holistic wellness journey.

Driven by a passion for uplifting others, Chris shares insights gained from years of motivating individuals towards positive change, integrating nutrition alongside mental health support, exercise routines, and environmental considerations. Embracing a holistic approach, Chris recognizes that true wellness encompasses nourishing the body, nurturing the mind, fostering physical activity, and creating a supportive environment conducive to growth and well-being. Through a blend of holistic practices, Chris guides individuals towards a balanced and fulfilling life, where nutrition serves as a cornerstone alongside other vital aspects of well-being.

For inquiries, speaking engagements, or collaboration opportunities, email: chriscooperbooks@gmail.com